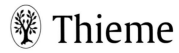

Atlas of Fundus Angiography

Heinrich Heimann, MD

Consultant Ophthalmic Surgeon
St. Paul's Eye Unit
Royal Liverpool University Hospital
Liverpool, United Kingdom

Ulrich Kellner, MD

Professor of Ophthalmology
AugenZentrum Siegburg
Siegburg, Germany
RetinaScience
Bonn, Germany

Michael H Foerster, MD

Professor of Ophthalmology
Department of Ophthalmology
Charité Campus Benjamin Franklin
Berlin, Germany

With contributions by
Nikolaos E Bechrakis, Jan Breckwoldt, Faik Gelisken,
Heinrich Heimann, Horst Helbig, Werner Inhoffen,
Claudia Jandeck, Ulrich Kellner, Lothar Krause,
Klaus-Martin Kreusel, Andreas Schueler, Joachim Wachtlin

Translated by Leslie Udvarhelyi

638 illustrations

Thieme
Stuttgart · New York

Library of Congress Cataloging-in-Publication Data is available from the publisher.

This book is an authorized and revised translation of the 1st German edition published and copyrighted 2004 by Georg Thieme Verlag, Stuttgart, Germany. Title of the German edition: Angiographie-Atlas des Augenhintergrundes.

Translator: Leslie Udvarhelyi, Universitäts Augenklinik, Charité Campus Benjamin Franklin, Berlin

© 2006 Georg Thieme Verlag,
Rüdigerstrasse 14, 70469 Stuttgart, Germany
http://www.thieme.de
Thieme New York, 333 Seventh Avenue,
New York, NY 10001, USA
http://www.thieme.com

Typesetting by primustype Hurler GmbH, Notzingen
Printed in Germany by Appl, Wemding

10-ISBN: 3-13-140551-1 (GTV)
13-ISBN: 978-3-13-140551-7 (GTV)
10-ISBN: 1-58890-438-5 (TNY)
13-ISBN: 978-1-58890-438-6 (TNY)   1 2 3 4 5 6

Dedication

This publication is dedicated to the memory of Professor Klaus Heimann (1935–1999), Director of the Department of Vitreoretinal Diseases at the University of Cologne, Germany (1975–1999)

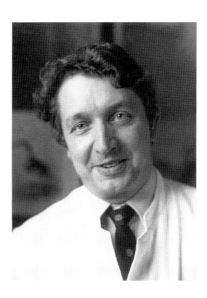

Preface

More than 40 years ago, the initial reports on fluorescein angiography of the ocular fundus were rejected by the major ophthalmology journals. In 1968, some 8 years after these pioneering works, Achim Wessing published the first German textbook on the subject. Since then, fluorescein angiography has become an established and standard examination technique in modern ophthalmology. The *Stereoscopic Atlas of Macular Diseases* by Donald Gass became the standard textbook for interpreting fluorescein-angiographic images.

Due to the procedure's low risk profile and a tendency for angiography to be misused as a method of documenting the course of diseases, fluorescein angiography has to some extent been overused in recent years. The landmark Early Treatment for Diabetic Retinopathy Study, providing a definition of "clinically significant macular edema," had already pointed out that angiography is only of value if a careful clinical examination has already raised a diagnostic or therapeutic question. The availability of new treatments for choroidal neovascularization (CNV) has more than doubled the number of angiographies carried out in tertiary centers in recent years. This in turn has led to increasing interest in the method of fluorescein angiography, as current treatment strategies and decision-making are largely based on the use of this technique as a "gold standard" for the classification of CNVs in accordance with the Macular Photocoagulation Study.

Apart from the advent of digital photography, the technical details of fluorescein angiography are still largely the same as the techniques described in the very first publications. Although stereoscopic techniques are necessary to differentiate the occult components of CNVs, this technique has not been met with widespread acceptance outside tertiary centers. Indocyanine angiography initially promised to become a new breakthrough technique for the diagnosis and treatment of choroid diseases in particular. However, following initial enthusiasm for the method, its use became limited to a few evidence-based indications. Optical coherence tomography is a noninvasive examination method that has clear advantages over fluorescein angiography with regard to the interpretation of diseases at the vitreoretinal interface and for qualitative and semiquantitative follow-up examinations of macular edema. However, it is not capable of replacing fluorescein angiography for treatment decision-making in the three most prevalent macular diseases encountered in everyday practice—age-related macular degeneration, diabetic macular edema, and retinal venous occlusions. The analysis of autofluorescence phenomena in the fundus promises to become one of the next examination methods that will come into use in routine clinical practice, particularly in nonexudative age-related macular degeneration and for early detection of hereditary retinal dystrophies and acquired retinal degeneration. The noninvasiveness of this method means that it has clear advantages over fluorescein angiography, but further evidence-based analysis of its value for clinical decision-making is still required in larger studies.

Following the success of a one-day course on fluorescein angiography held annually in Berlin before the German Ophthalmological Society Conference, we asked the course lecturers, from various departments in Germany and Switzerland, to convert their thorough lectures and excellent images into concise chapters for this textbook. Every effort has been made to bridge the gap between the interpretation of angiograms and decision-making in a clinical setting, and to separate evidence-based indications for angiography from those of more academic interest. The typical angiographic findings in the most prevalent diseases are therefore shown here along with essential information regarding the pathogenesis, the causes of the angiographic phenomena, and implications for treatment. The aim of the book is to provide a compact guide for the beginner as well as for the more advanced clinician.

The majority of the images were taken by highly skilled and specialized photographers, particularly Gesa Bröskamp and Karin Ehrenberg (Berlin), Hugo Niederberger (St. Gallen), Ernst Kleinknecht, Susanne Schweyer, and Anette Keck (Tübingen) and Silke Weinitz (Siegburg). The autofluorescence images were provided by Agnes B. Renner and Hilmar Tillack (Berlin) and Silke Weinitz (Siegburg). We would also like to express our gratitude to all of the staff in the participating departments who were involved in the treatment of the patients. Particular thanks are also due to Antje-Karen Richter, Mona Chatterjee, and Elke Plach at Thieme Medical Publishers, who helped us put together the first edition of this book.

Following the success of the first German edition of the atlas, it was soon decided to translate it into English. All of the chapters were revised by the individual authors and editors, and new information was included—e.g., new treatment strategies for age-related macular disease and the use of infrared reflectance imaging and fundus autofluorescence in macular disease—as well as a large number of new images. All of the reference lists were also updated. We would like to thank Leslie Udvarhelyi for the careful translation of the German text and Annie Hollins and Cliff Bergman at Thieme Medical Publishers for their support in the preparation of this English edition.

Last but not least, we would like to thank all of the contributing authors for the dedication and care they have put into preparing their chapters.

Heinrich Heimann
Ulrich Kellner
Michael Foerster

Contributors

Nikolaos E Bechrakis, MD
Professor of Ophthalmology
Department of Ophthalmology
Charité Campus Benjamin Franklin
Berlin, Germany

Jan Breckwoldt, MD
Department of Anesthesiology
Charité Campus Benjamin Franklin
Berlin, Germany

Michael H Foerster, MD
Professor of Ophthalmology
Department of Ophthalmology
Charité Campus Benjamin Franklin
Berlin, Germany

Faik Gelisken, MD
Department of Ophthalmology I
University of Tuebingen
Tuebingen, Germany

Heinrich Heimann, MD
Consultant Ophthalmic Surgeon
St. Paul's Eye Unit
Royal Liverpool University Hospital
Liverpool, United Kingdom

Horst Helbig, MD
Professor of Ophthalmology
Universitaetsspital Zurich
Zurich, Switzerland

Werner Inhoffen, DSc
Department of Ophthalmology I
University of Tuebingen
Tuebingen, Germany

Claudia Jandeck, MD
Associate Professor of Ophthalmology
Artemis Zentren Dillenburg/Frankfurt
Dillenburg, Germany

Ulrich Kellner, MD
Professor of Ophthalmology
AugenZentrum Siegburg
Siegburg, Germany
RetinaScience
Bonn, Germany

Lothar Krause, MD
Department of Ophthalmology
Charité Campus Benjamin Franklin
Berlin, Germany

Klaus-Martin Kreusel, MD
Associate Professor of Ophthalmology
Eye Center
DRK-Kliniken Westend
Berlin, Germany

Andreas Schueler, MD
Eye Clinic Universitaetsallee
Bremen, Germany

Joachim Wachtlin, MD
Associate Professor of Ophthalmology
Charité Campus Benjamin Franklin
Berlin, Germany

Contents

1.1 Fluorescein Angiography   *Heinrich Heimann*

Fluorescence and Fluorescein Angiography

- The term "fluorescence" refers to solid, liquid, or gaseous matter that emits absorbed radiated energy in the form of electromagnetic radiation at similar or longer wavelengths.
- In fluorescence angiography, a fluorescent substance is administered intravenously; shortly afterwards, it spreads through the choroid via the bloodstream and retinal vessels. Stimulating light enters the eye through a filter and then, as a result of the substance's fluorescence, produces light emission at varying wavelengths, which are reduced to appropriately defined emission spectra through a second filter; these can then be photographed and/or filmed.
- Two different intravenous fluorescent substances are currently in use in ophthalmology: fluorescein and indocyanine green. The two substances differ in their absorption and emission spectra, in their pharmacological characteristics (particularly their binding properties to plasma proteins) and in their elimination and passage through vascular walls in the choroid and retina.
- The development of the methodology and the clinical applications of fluorescein angiography are based on the work of Chao and Flocks, Novotny and Alvis, and MacLean and Maumenee. These angiographic methods have been in regular use for retinal diagnosis since the 1960s. In Germany, fluorescein angiography was first introduced, developed, and popularized by Wessing.

Sodium Fluorescein

- Sodium fluorescein ($C_{20}H_{10}O_5Na_2$, MG 376) is the dye most commonly used for fluorescence angiography throughout the world. After agitation, the fluorescence lasts for 10^{-9} seconds (there is therefore no "afterglow" as in phosphorescent substances).
- Both the absorption and emission spectra of sodium fluorescein depend on various factors; with intravenous administration, they are 465 nm (absorption) and 525 nm (emission).
- Approximately 70–80% of the sodium fluorescein binds to plasma proteins; 20–30% does not bind. Injected fluorescein is diluted in the bloodstream by a factor of approximately 600 and disperses throughout the whole body. With the exception of the central nervous system vessels, the retina, and to a limited extent the iris, unbound sodium fluorescein can freely permeate all blood vessels in the body. A few minutes after injection, the skin, mucosa (visible up to 6 h after injection), and urine (visible up to 36 h after injection, or longer if kidney function is limited) show signs of the yellow dye. Some laboratory values can be affected until the dye is completely eliminated from the body. The elimination of sodium fluorescein predominantly takes place through the kidney rather than the liver.

- **Contraindications:**
  - Known hypersensitivity to fluorescein derivatives. Some companies specify that beta-blocker treatment is a contraindication. Beta-blockers do not interact with fluorescein directly, but allergic reactions are more difficult to treat.
  - There are no medically established contraindications in pregnancy. Despite this, the examination is carried out in pregnant women only in exceptional circumstances.
  - Sodium fluorescein has some limited vasoconstrictive and photosensitizing characteristics (skin irritation by sunlight after injection); however, these are not considered to be serious or significant.

Prerequisites for Fluorescein Angiography

- Despite evidence of very good general tolerance of injected sodium fluorescein, the physician administering or supervising the treatment should be adequately trained in emergency procedures. Medication required during an emergency must be administered reliably and without delay. Immediate notification of the need for emergency care and implementation of it must be ensured (see Chapter 2).
- Secure intravenous access is important; if extravascular or intra-arterial injection take place, severe side effects such as skin necrosis or intense yellow discoloring of the surrounding skin can be expected. Intravenous access should be maintained until the examination has been completed.
- The following equipment is essential: a fundus camera with automatic film transport, or a digital camera; an electronic flash unit with an exciter filter of 465–490 nm (the blue–green spectrum); and a recording filter of 520–530 nm (the green–yellow spectrum). Enlargement and editing of images for retinal analysis can be carried out (depending on the type of fundus camera used) using the various sizes of field available. A standard exposure setting of 30° for macular diseases is routinely used; in addition, 20° (the largest enlargement possible with a small section) and 50° or 60° exposures are also used.
- Photographic documentation of the filtered, emitted light is recorded on highly sensitive black-and-white film, or in electronic image files with a digital camera system. Newer scanning laser ophthalmoscopes (SLOs) are also usually equipped to handle fluorescein angiography. Digital documentation systems have been increasingly used in practice in recent years. These have the advantages of allowing immediate assessment and editing of the images (with adjustment of contrast and brilliance) and also of providing electronic archiving and data storage, enabling fast computer-networked access to the data from several locations.
- At present, however, film documentation still provides higher resolution. In private practices and most clinical

centres, digital technology has established itself as the main examination method.

- Experience and knowledge on the part of the photographer, along with cooperation by the patient, determine the quality of the images taken for analysis. Other factors that can have a negative effect on the quality of an angiogram are: clouding of the media; insufficient pupil dilation; too slow or insufficient injection of dye; and unreliable or badly configured equipment or faulty processing of the angiograms.

Practical Procedure

- Before angiography is started, it is recommended to take a color exposure and a blank black-and-white exposure of the fundus. There should always be clarity about the structures to be examined, any potentially important phase of the angiography to be observed, and the enlargement chosen. Photographic documentation of the findings in the second eye should also be obtained in order to allow comparisons with the eye being treated and for monitoring.
- Angiography starts with an intravenous bolus administration of 5 ml 10% sodium fluorescein solution (equivalent to 500 mg active agent; today's commercially available compounds usually come in ready-made solution vials). For patients with renal insufficiency, a reduced dose of 2.5 ml of the appropriate solution is recommended. A stopwatch should be used during the injection in order to plot the chronology of the exposures.
- Inflow of dye into the choroidal vessels can usually be seen after 10–15 s; this is directly followed by the retinal circulation. Experienced photographers can "anticipate" the inflow of the dye and immediately start taking sequential exposures. The fast arterial and arteriovenous phase of the angiography which then follows places very high demands on the photographer, who has to take sequential exposures (starting with approximately one image per second) within a very short period of time, continuing until the maximum fluorescence is reached (this is usually 25–35 s after the start of the angiography). Angiography is concluded with the last exposures being taken 5, 10, or 15 min after the initial injection. The protocols used at different institutions vary depending on the profile of the disease and the institution carrying out the angiography.
- After completion of the arteriovenous phase, additional exposures of the fundus periphery (for example, in diabetic retinopathy) or the second eye (for example, in macular degeneration) should be made in accordance with the diagnosed profile of the disease. Parallel complete angiography of both eyes is not possible with standard equipment.
- After completion of the angiography, six to eight typical exposures (determined by the analysis technique used) of the individual phases of the angiography should be selected and enlarged—or, where applicable (digital angiography), digitally processed and saved for documentation purposes—and printed out. Storage of all unenlarged negatives—in other words, complete picture data—is recommended in all cases.

- In situations in which the resulting images are inadequate for interpretation, the angiography can be repeated in most diseases after 2 h, at which time no fluorescence phenomena can usually be detected in the choroid vessels or in the retina. However, in larger studies, a 48-h interval is generally recommended.
- Using the appropriate equipment, fluorescein angiography and indocyanine green angiography can be carried out, either in parallel or shortly after each other. Mutual interference between the fluorescence phenomena displayed does not occur, although some investigators have reported an increase in side effects during simultaneous angiography.

Interpretation

- The interpretation of fluorescein angiography is a subjective method that is influenced by the timing of individual exposures, their quality, the actual exposures chosen for analysis, the way in which the picture is viewed, and finally the experience and qualification of the investigator. Interobserver and intraobserver differences in the interpretation of fluorescein angiography can occur.
- When in doubt, cases should be discussed with an experienced colleague; with the advent of digital angiography and the internet, this has become a fast and relatively simple procedure.
- The analysis and diagnosis of angiographies are carried out in different ways. Technically, the best method is analyzing stereo angiography (see section 1.4). Another alternative is the single enlargement of a 35-mm film angiogram or monitor image, which can also be appropriately printed out for consultation purposes. Selection, modification and printout of single images should be carried out by the investigator or an experienced photographer in a standardized way. In any case, storage of all unedited pictures taken during angiography is advisable.
- For interpretation, the following patient information is important: medical history; course of the disease; previous treatment; visual acuity; and concomitant diagnosis.
- The clinical diagnosis should be known to the consultant, who should at least receive a color image. Color images help identify structures that may be hard to define with angiography alone.
- The availability of previous angiograms is helpful for monitoring purposes—for example, relating to the enlargement or reduction of a choroidal neovascularization after treatment.
- During interpretation, the examiner determines whether the angiographic findings are normal and allocates them spatially (anatomical structures) and chronologically (early, middle, or late phase of the angiography). Ideally, diagnosis and the resulting treatment are based on a combination of the clinical findings and angiographic findings.

Avoiding Unnecessary Angiographies

- Like all diagnostic procedures, fluorescein angiography is used to diagnose conditions in order to determine the need for therapeutic procedures and to follow up specific diseases.
- Despite good tolerance and high levels of safety, fluorescein angiography is still an invasive procedure that can potentially lead to serious side effects. Unnecessary angiography should therefore be avoided.
- Angiography should not be performed if a diagnosis can be made without it or if no therapeutic consequences would result from the procedure. Angiography is also unsuitable as a method of routine check-up or for documentation purposes—for example, in the course of a diabetic macular edema or macular degeneration.
- In our experience, numerous unnecessary angiographies are often carried out in the following groups of diseases in particular:
  - Age-related macular degeneration in unique clinical diagnosis without therapeutic consequences (for example, disciform scarring or geographic atrophy, dry and atrophic scarring after photodynamic therapy).
  - Diabetic retinopathy for the diagnosis of a clinically significant macular edema or as a "routine check-up."
  - Unexplained loss of visual acuity in a clinically normal-appearing macula; no additional information can be expected from angiography.
  - Choroidal melanoma. Angiography provides little additional information in cases of suspected choroidal melanoma.
  - Occlusion of retinal vessels. The diagnosis can usually be established without angiography. Reliable conclusions regarding treatment can only be made in cases of vein occlusions, and then usually only months after vessel occlusion. It is debatable whether angiography can determine the necessity of panretinal laser coagulation following retinal vein occlusion.
  - Hereditary retinal dystrophies. Fundus autofluorescence usually provides sufficient information, even earlier or in more detail than fluorescein angiography, which is only appropriate when exudative complications are expected.

Normal Fluorescein Angiography

- Blood flow in the choroidal and retinal vessels can be visualized using fluorescein angiography. After injection into a peripheral vein, the sodium fluorescein reaches the vascular system in the eye via the blood circulation system and the central retinal artery. Sodium fluorescein diffuses quickly within the fluid compartments of the eye, but it does not usually pass through the retinal vessels and the retinal pigment epithelium (RPE). Fluorescein angiography therefore examines the integrity of the blood–retina barrier.
- Two vessel systems, the choroidal vessel system and the retinal vessel system, with differing degrees of extravasation of fluorescein, fill almost simultaneously. These are separated by the RPE. Due to the presence of tight junctions, fluorescein is virtually incapable of permeating the vascular walls (the internal blood–retina barrier) of normal retinal vessels and large choroidal vessels. The dye freely permeates the fenestrated vessels of the choriocapillaris and spreads very rapidly within the choroid.
- As well as acting as an optical barrier to stimulating and emitting light, the RPE also acts as a barrier against fluorescein, because of its zonula occludens. The pigment content of the RPE in patients of African or Asian descent is comparable to that of less pigmented races. The difference between the lightness of the background of the eye is based on the variable pigmentation within the choroid.
- The first visible change is that the choriocapillaris of the choroid is filled via the posterior ciliary arteries. The flooding of the fluorescein relates to the lobular structure of the choriocapillaris. Although there is no immediately visible barrier, interindividually variable segment-shaped filling of the choriocapillaris is noticeable. In the periphery, these patches resemble spindle-type segments. The long posterior ciliary arteries fill a nasal and temporal segment. Early choroidal vessel filling is only of diagnostic significance in particular lesions (for example, choroidal hemangioma) or when there is patchy and delayed filling (for example, in anterior ischemic optic neuropathy or ocular ischemic syndrome).
- Cilioretinal vessels may fill at the same time as the choriocapillaris and, as a rule, slightly earlier than the actual retinal vessels.
- The first signs of the dye in the retinal vessels can be seen 10–15 s after the start of the injection (known as the "arm–retina time" and averaging about 11 s in healthy young individuals). Filling of the retinal vessels takes place 0–2 s after filling of the choroidal vessels. The arteriovenous passage time (the time between the first signs of the dye in the arteries close to the optic nerve head and the first signs in the veins) averages 1.5 s. Another definition of the arteriovenous passage time is the time span between the first signs of the dye in the temporal arteries and complete filling of the large temporal retinal veins (normal value up to 11 s).
- The retinal vessels are located in the inner two-thirds of the retina; the outer third, incorporating the photoreceptors, is vessel-free. The arterial branches represent end arteries without anastomoses. The retinal arteries and veins course in the ganglion cell layer; the capillaries form deep, extensive interweaving layers that reach the outer plexiform layer. A distinguished surface capillary layer is visible in the peripapillary area.
- After injection, the dye spreads into the central retinal artery and into the retinal arteries, initially with an axial flow. The unbound fluorescein in particular is visible, which in practice represents the plasma flow. Since the column of erythrocytes in the blood vessels is seen in normal fundus images, the vessels appear comparatively wider on fluorescein angiography. Stronger fluorescence is noticeable in anemic patients due to the relatively high plasma content.
- All arterial branches are filled within one or two seconds, after which transit into the capillary area, fol-

lowed by the macula area, can be observed. The orientation and density of the capillary network shows regional variations (macula, optic nerve head, periphery). Due to their high xanthophyll concentration and increased pigmentation resulting from blockage of choroidal fluorescence, the central macular areas appear darker.

- Simultaneously with the filling of the arteries in the fundus periphery, filling of the retinal veins also starts in the retina. As the fluorescein arrives in the central venules prior to the peripheral venules in the efferent veins, laminar flow can be seen in the vessels. Approximately 25 s later, the dye is evenly distributed in the arteries and veins; at this point, the perifoveal capillary network can be seen best. After reaching a maximum concentration level, the visible intraluminal fluorescence in the retinal vessel decreases.
- In the meantime, the dye leaves the fenestrated vessels of the choriocapillaris within a few seconds and diffuses into the choroidal tissue, resulting in a relatively homogeneous background fluorescence that reaches its climax more or less parallel to the filling of the retinal capillaries. Subsequently, the fluorescein molecules in the choroidal vessel follow a corresponding concentration gradient (by diffusion) back into the vessel. As a result of dilution and elimination, the background fluorescein decreases.
- Both the posterior ciliary arteries and numerous retinal capillaries are visible on the optic nerve head, resulting in distinct coloring of the optic disc during the course of the angiography. A low-grade leakage phenomenon can also be encountered in the optic disc area as a result of the fenestrated peripapillary choriocapillaris and staining of the lamina cribrosa in normal angiograms.
- The last phenomenon in fluorescein angiography is staining of the inner scleral layers, which is visible as a result of contrast with the choroidal vessels.
- There is no standardized pattern for describing the various phases of angiography; individual interpretations and arbitrary classifications are used. In general, however, a distinction is made between an early phase (the filling of the retinal arteries or "arterial phase"); a middle phase or arteriovenous phase (the arteriovenous transition, often further subdivided into early, middle and late arteriovenous phases); and a late phase (in which the fluorescein angiographic phenomena decline). The timing of the late phase is handled in a variety of ways; usually, an exposure is carried out after 5 min. In specific diseases (for example, distinct leakage or staining in exudative macular degeneration), exposure after 10 min is necessary.

Identifying Abnormal Appearances in Fluorescein Angiography

- The interpretation of fluorescein angiography is based on the identification of fluorescein phenomena that differ from those in normal angiography. These aspects are placed in a spatial and chronological context and are compared with known changes in specific diseases.
- Angiographic phenomena that differ from those of normal angiography can be divided into two groups: hyperfluorescence and hypofluorescence. Hyperfluorescence means added fluorescein detection in comparison with normal angiography. Leakage shows the transfer of fluorescein into the surrounding tissue, usually from permeable vessels. Hypofluorescence, in contrast, means weaker fluorescein detection in comparison with normal angiography.
- The causes of hyperfluorescence and hypofluorescence are numerous. Furthermore, both hyperfluorescence and hypofluorescence can occur in various combinations within one and the same angiographic examination.
- Hyperfluorescence and hypofluorescence should always be interpreted according to the anatomic structural relationship, the phases of angiography, and the possible changes during the course of angiography. Consequently, early-phase hyperfluorescence can become late-phase hypofluorescence and vice versa.

Hyperfluorescence

- Hyperfluorescence can arise in what are known as "window defects," in newly formed vessels, in vessel-conducting structures, or due to dysfunction of the inner or outer blood–retina barrier.
- In window defects, increased visibility of the normal choroidal vessel fluorescence takes place because of a defect in the RPE. An early sharply demarcated hyperfluorescence that decreases in the subsequent course is typical. Leakage phenomena (with the hyperfluorescence spreading like the smudging of watercolor paint) are not encountered.
- In newly formed vessels or vessel-conducting structures, hyperfluorescence arises from their location, also producing additional fluorescence in the corresponding anatomical structures. In addition, newly formed vessels are usually more permeable to unbound fluorescein. Early hyperfluorescence as a result of filling of the newly formed vessels in the arterial phase followed by an increase in the subsequent course as a result of leakage is typical. In contrast to neovascularization, collateral formation typically shows weaker leakage phenomena.
- Damage to the external blood–retina barrier caused by functional changes in the RPE is visible mostly in the form of late hyperfluorescence, through an accumulation of the dye in front or behind the RPE (for example, in central serous chorioretinopathy).
- Damage to the inner blood–retina barrier mainly results in extravascular and increasing hyperfluorescence with leakage phenomena (for example, in retinal vasculitis).

Hypofluorescence

- Hypofluorescence occurs as a result of a decrease in the stimulating or emitting light or the dye-conducting structures.
- Classically, hypofluorescence occurs due to the blockage of normal fluorescence (for example, "exclusion" of the stimulating light and occlusion of the choroidal fluorescence as a result of retinal hemorrhage), or as a

result of reduced perfusion (for example, in arterial occlusion).

- The transition from initial hypofluorescence to subsequent hyperfluorescence can typically be observed in inflammatory changes both to the retina and to the choroidal vessel, and in specific tumor-like changes. The initial hypofluorescence is explained by blockage phenomena (for example, in retinal edema or tumor), followed by a hyperfluorescence as a result of added vessels or more permeable vessels within these structures.

References

Bloom JN, Herman DC, Elin RJ, et al. Intravenous fluorescein interference with clinical laboratory tests. Am J Ophthalmol 1989;108: 375–9.

Halperin LS, Olk RJ, Soubrane G, Coscas G. Safety of fluorescein angiography during pregnancy. Am J Ophthalmol 1990;109:563–6.

Holz FG, Jorzik J, Schutt F, Flach U, Unnebrink K. Agreement among ophthalmologists in evaluating fluorescein angiograms in patients with neovascular age-related macular degeneration for photodynamic therapy eligibility (FLAP-study). Ophthalmology 2003;110:400–5.

Wessing A. Fluoreszenzangiografie der Retina. Lehrbuch und Atlas. Stuttgart: Thieme, 1968.

Wolf S, Arend O, Reim M. Measurement of retinal hemodynamics with scanning laser ophthalmoscopy: reference values and variation. Surv Ophthalmol 1994;38:95–100.

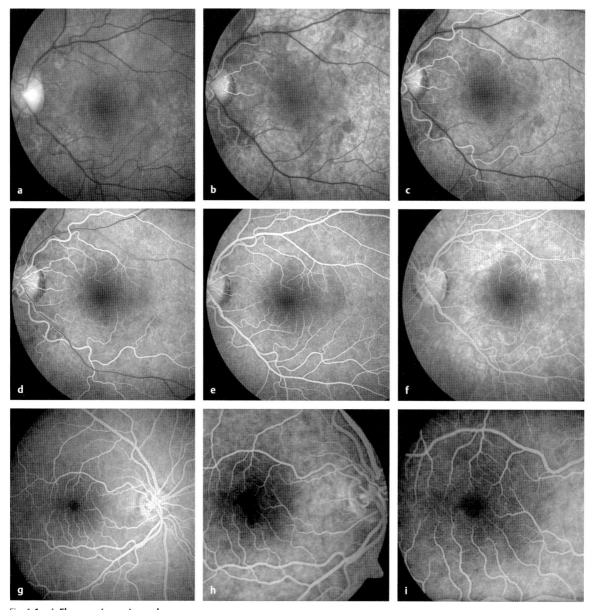

Fig. 1.1a–i Fluorescein angiography

a The first phenomenon observed in fluorescein angiography is filling of the choroidal vessel. The retinal vessels have not yet filled with fluorescein here (13 s after injection).

b Early arterial phase. The retinal arteries are starting to fill with fluorescein. The choroidal vessel dye is spreading further and is already starting to diffuse (16 s).

c Early arteriovenous phase. The retinal veins close to the optic nerve head show laminar filling; there is still no dye recognizable in the peripheral veins. With its higher pigment content, the central macula masks the choroidal vessel fluorescein, and as a result looks darker (17 s).

d Middle arteriovenous phase. Laminar flow is recognizable in the main stems of the retinal veins. (19 s).

e Late arteriovenous phase. The dye has homogenously spread in the arteries and veins. The parafoveal capillaries are at their best visibility in this phase. The choroid is also homogenously filled;

rediffusion of the fluorescein into the choroidal vessel is starting (31 s).

f Late phase. The fluorescein angiographic phenomena are decreasing; the dye is still faintly recognizable in the retinal vessels. The choroidal vessels appear as a shadow against the still-active fluorescein in the sclera (5 min).

g Image with a 50° section, providing a good overview from the retina to the vessel arcades.

h This image with a 30° section shows the macula and optic nerve with good resolution. The 30° image is the standard for the majority of angiographies carried out.

i Image with a 20° section. This allows even more detail to be shown. However, sharp focus is more difficult to achieve and the smaller section means that the optic nerve and the macula cannot be displayed simultaneously and are more likely to be out of focus.

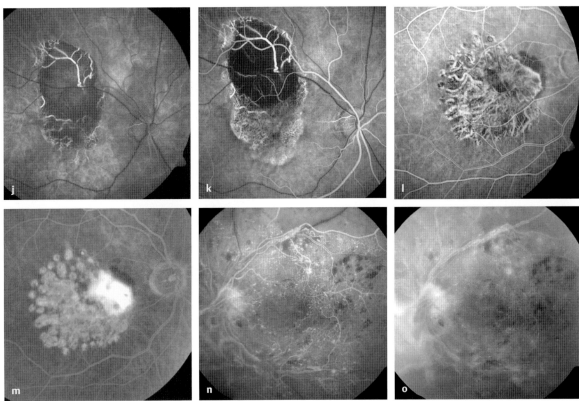

Fig. 1.1j–o Fluorescein angiography

j Early phase, showing the various vessel systems in a patient after surgical extraction of an idiopathic choroidal neovascularization, where a part of the choroid, the choriocapillaris, and the retinal pigment epithelium (RPE) have been removed. Before filling of the retinal vessels takes place, filling of the large choroidal vessel is recognizable in the depth of the lesion. Like retinal vessels, these large choroidal vessels do not leak fluorescein. As a result of the absent RPE, these vessels are easier to see (hyperfluorescence as a result of a "window defect").

k Early arteriovenous phase. The choriocapillaris is absent from the upper part of the lesion; the absence of this layer of tissue results in hypofluorescence. The choriocapillaris is still present on the lower edge of the lesion, but the RPE is absent in places. The distribution of the fluorescein into the individual choroidal vessels is visible here. Outside the lesion, the effects of choroidal filling are less distinct due to masking by the RPE.

l Various causes of hyperfluorescence in macular degeneration. In the temporal part of the lesion, geographic atrophy with a defect in the RPE has developed; hyperfluorescence forms here as a result of a window-defect and better visibility of the choroidal vessels. Choroidal neovascularization has developed in the central section, which fills with the dye from the earlier arteriovenous phase.

m In the late phase, the hyperfluorescence is sharply delimited in the temporal area as a result of the window defect. Leakage (continuation of hyperfluorescence beyond the border of the original hyperfluorescence) can be observed in the nasal region, in the area of the neovascularization. Above the neovascularization, a blockage in an area of subretinal hemorrhage is visible in all phases of the angiography.

n Various areas of hyperfluorescence and hypofluorescence in proliferative diabetic retinopathy (early arteriovenous phase). In the upper part of the image, hypofluorescence as a result of hyperpigmentation after laser coagulation, reduced perfusion in capillary occlusions, and intraretinal hemorrhage can be seen. Areas of hyperfluorescence as a result of microaneurysms, intraretinal vessel anomalies, and vessel proliferation can also be seen.

o In the late phase, clear leakage is visible over the neovascularization of the optic disc and above the fovea. The collaterals and microaneurysm show fewer leakage phenomena in the late phases. As a result of damage to the vessel walls, the wall of the main vein stem of the upper vascular arcade shows persistent staining. Hypofluorescence in the area of the laser focus, bleeding, and areas of reduced perfusion persist.

1.2 Indocyanine Green Angiography   *Faik Gelisken*

Indocyanine Green

- Indocyanine green (ICG) is a water-soluble tricarbocyanine dye with a molecular weight of 774.96 Da.
- Due to the excitation and emission spectrum in the infrared range (780–810 nm), ICG angiography produces better transmission through hemorrhages, pigmentation, and exudations in comparison with fluorescein angiography.
- Ninety-eight percent of the ICG dye binds to plasma proteins, and resulting in a lower level of leakage in comparison with fluorescein dye.
- Because of the differences between ICG and fluorescein angiography, ICG angiography is advantageous for the analysis of the choroidal vessel structure.
- ICG angiography is generally well tolerated (better than fluorescein). Nausea and vomiting seldom occur. However, a few life-threatening incidents have been reported (see Chapter 2).
- The side effects of ICG mainly depend on the iodine used to stabilize the dye.
- **Contraindications to ICG angiography:**
  - Allergy to ICG or iodine and decompensated liver disease. In patients who are allergic to iodine, ICG angiography can be carried out (if clinically necessary) using iodine-free compounds.
  - Hyperthyroidism (if clinically necessary, after consultation with an internist).
  - ICG angiography is not recommended during pregnancy.

Procedure

- Before the start of the examination, a blank image should be taken to detect any possible pseudohyperfluorescence. A bolus of 25–50 mg ICG dye solution should then be injected intravenously.
- Several images should be taken within the first minute. Thereafter, images should be taken every minute for 5 min, with further images taken after 10, 20, and 30 min.
- Various angiography systems can be used for ICG angiography: the scanning laser ophthalmoscope (SLO; Rodenstock, Germany); confocal SLO (HRA; Heidelberg Engineering, Germany); and fundus camera-supported systems (e. g., Topcon, Japan, Zeiss, Germany).
- SLO and confocal SLO are better suited for dynamic analysis of subretinal vessels (anastomoses between retinal vessels and choroidal neovascularization).
- Fundus camera-supported systems provide better-quality imaging of peripheral lesions and more detail in the later phases.
- As the various imaging systems in some cases produce different types of images for the same findings, interpretation is more difficult and more subjective with ICG angiography than with fluorescein angiography.

Phases of Indocyanine Green Angiography

1—Early phase
- The choroidal arteries, choriocapillaris, and veins fill a few seconds after the indocyanine green reaches the choroid circulation.

2—Middle phase (late venous phase)
- There is a slow decrease in the contrast between the choroidal vessels and the background, with isofluorescence at the end of the phase. Duration: 10–20 min.

3—Late Phase (inversion phase)
- Dark visible choroidal vessels appear against the homogeneous background fluorescence. This phase starts 10–15 min after injection of the ICG dye.

Interpretation of Indocyanine Green Angiography

- The logic of interpreting ICG angiography is similar to that of fluorescein angiography, with a few important differences:
  - Due to the transmission of infrared light, there is no blockage of the retinal pigment epithelium (RPE). When the choriocapillaris is intact, therefore, there is only relative hyperfluorescence in the absent of pigment epithelium area.
- Hyperfluorescence caused by leakage is better delimited than with fluorescein angiography due to the high level of binding to plasma proteins, resulting in a slower leakage of the ICG dye.

Causes of Hypofluorescence

- Blockage can result from pigment, subretinal fluid, or hemorrhage (despite better transmission of infrared light, the penetration depth depends on the density of these lesions).
- Filling defects can result from atrophy or perfusion dysfunction of the choroid (previous laser coagulation, photodynamic therapy, inflammation, malignant arterial hypertension).

Causes of Hyperfluorescence

- Leakage can arise from pathological vessels (choroidal neovascularization) or hyperpermeability of the choroid (central serous chorioretinopathy).
- Staining of fibrin, Bruch membrane, or the retinal pigment epithelium.
- Pseudohyperfluorescence (hyperfluorescence before the injection of ICG dye) can be seen in the presence of old organized subretinal hemorrhage, lipofuscin, pigmented choroidal neovascularization, or chronic central serous chorioretinopathy.

Artefacts

- "Blooming effect." Hyperfluorescence that is often seen in the retinal filling phase as a result of the higher light intensity of fundus camera-supported systems.
- Cross-over of the choroidal vessels can cause focal hyperfluorescence.

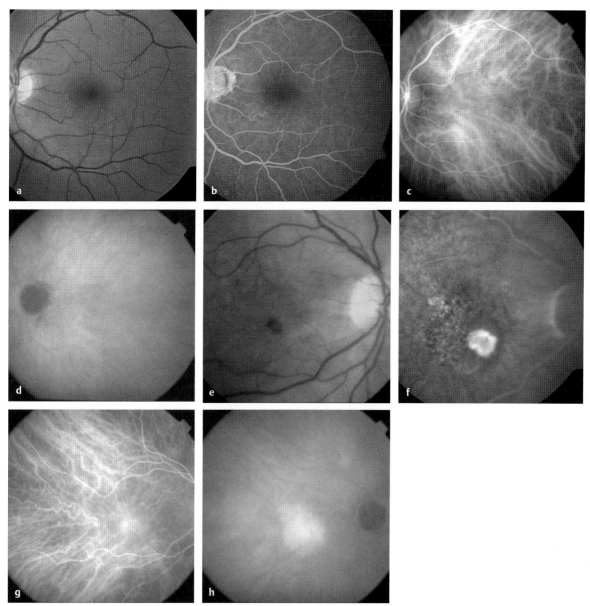

Fig. 1.2a–d Normal findings

a Color photograph. A homogeneous distribution of the pigment is visible at the posterior pole. The dark reflex in the fovea is due to xanthophyll pigment.

b Arteriovenous phase of fluorescein angiography. A homogeneous background fluorescence is visible. The background fluorescence results from choroidal fluorescence and the blockage effect of the retinal pigment epithelium (RPE). Temporal to the optic disc is a "window defect" caused by atrophy of the RPE. Hypofluorescence in the fovea is caused by blockage of the xanthophyll pigment.

c Middle phase of indocyanine green (ICG) angiography. The choroidal vessels are visible. The blockage effect of the normal RPE is not visible due to the penetration of infrared light. Because of this characteristic, the high contrast between the retinal vessel and the background is lacking in ICG angiography.

d Late phase of ICG angiography. Thirty minutes after the injection of ICG, homogenous fluorescence (isofluorescence) is visible at the fundus. The optic nerve can be seen as a hypofluorescent round structure. The dark silhouettes of the large choroidal vessels can be seen.

Fig. 1.2e–h Hyperfluorescence

e Color photograph. Macular edema and subretinal hemorrhage are visible in the nasal area in the right eye, inferior to the fovea.

f Fluorescein angiography. In the early phase, a bright hyperfluorescent structure consistent with a classic choroidal neovascularization can be seen.

g Middle phase of indocyanine green angiography. The network of the choroidal neovascularization is visible in the fovea. The pathological vessels in the choroidal neovascularization are visible for longer than in fluorescein angiography, because of slow leakage.

h Late phase of indocyanine green angiography. Subfoveal hyperfluorescence caused by leakage from the classic choroidal neovascularization.

- Blurred images may occur in the late phase in ICG angiography due to a high exposure setting in SLO.

Indications

- ICG angiography can provide information additional to that offered by fluorescein angiography. The differences have been observed and described in recent years mainly in scientific research studies. Due to the greater expense of the equipment, ICG angiography is not as widely used as fluorescein angiography. Outside of research studies, the use of ICG angiography in everyday clinical practice is limited to specific diseases:
  - Differentiating between subgroups of age-related neovascular macular degeneration: retinal angiomatosis proliferation, chorioretinal anastomosis, and polypoidal choroidal vasculopathy.
  - The differential diagnosis of central serous chorioretinopathy.
  - Inflammation of the choroid.
  - Epiretinal hemorrhage: for accurate diagnosis of arterial macroaneurysms or retinal angiomatosis proliferation.
  - Differential diagnosis of amelanotic flat fundus lesions (choroidal hemangioma).

References

Bischoff PM, Flower RW. Ten years experience with choroid angiography using indocyanine green dye: a new routine examination or an epilogue? Doc Opthalmol 1985;60:235–91.

Hope-Ross M, Yannuzzi LA, Gragoudas ES, et al. Adverse reactions due to indocyanine green. Ophthalmology 1994;101:529–33.

Soubrane G, Seres A, Coscas G, Flower RW. Suggested terminology for different phases of indocyanine green angiogram. Retina 2000;20:319–20.

Stanga PE, Lim JI, Hamilton P. Indocyanine green angiography in chorioretinal diseases: indications and interpretation: an evidence-based update. Ophthalmology 2003;110:15–21.

Yannuzzi LA, Flower RW, Slakter JS, eds. Indocyanine green angiography. St. Louis: Mosby, 1997.

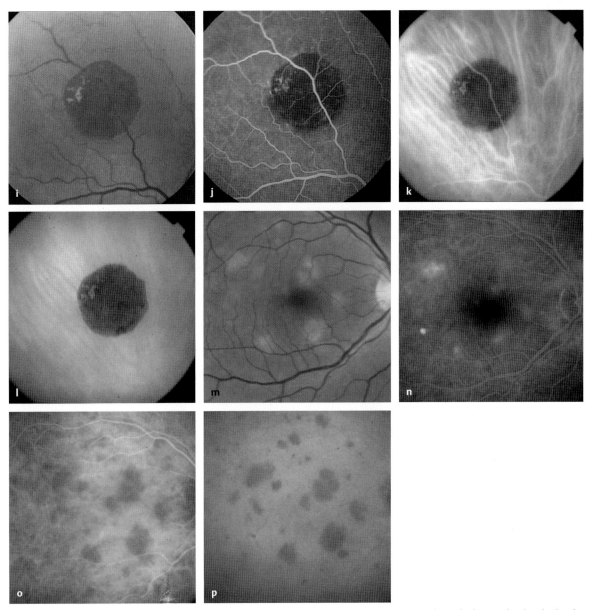

Fig. 1.2i–p Hypofluorescence

i Color photograph. A darkly pigmented flat subretinal lesion is visible in the periphery of the right eye, resembling congenital hypertrophy of the retinal pigment epithelium.

j Fluorescein angiography. In the arteriovenous phase, hypofluorescence caused by blockage of the pigmented fundus lesion is visible.

k Middle phase of indocyanine green angiography. The choroidal vessels are visible in the late venous phase. The normal retinal pigment epithelium did not produce a blockage effect, but the lesion caused hypofluorescence. This hypofluorescence, arising from heavy pigmentation, is the result of a blockage effect (in the same way as in fluorescein angiography).

l Late phase of indocyanine green angiography. The washing out of the ICG dye leads to isofluorescence of the fundus. The dark silhouettes of the large choroidal vessels are recognizable. The hypofluorescent lesion is also unchanged in the late phase.

m Color photograph. Perimacular multiple, round and oval, whitish–yellowish subretinal lesions can be seen in the right eye. The finding is consistent with acute posterior multifocal placoid pigment epitheliopathy (see section 9.7).

n Late phase of fluorescein angiography. Multiple areas of hyperfluorescence are visible at the posterior pole.

o Middle phase of indocyanine green (ICG) angiography. Multiple hypofluorescent lesions can be seen at the posterior pole 20 s after ICG administration.

p Late phase of ICG angiography. Persistence of the hypofluorescence is detectable in the late phase. The hypofluorescence is consistent with filling defects, caused by occlusion of the choriocapillaris.

1.3 Fundus Autofluorescence   *Ulrich Kellner*

Basic Physiological and Morphological Principles

- Lifelong phagocytosis of the photoreceptor outer segment takes place in the lysosomes of retinal pigment epithelium (RPE) cells. In healthy eyes, the majority of the resultant end products are transported away from the cells toward the choroid via the basal membrane. With increasing age, the amount of degradation product that remains in the lipofuscin granula of the RPE cells increases. A disturbance of the phagocytotic process in the RPE cells or increased shedding of outer segments are possible mechanisms underlying alteration of the lipofuscin content in various diseases.
- There are various degradation products in the lipofuscin granula, at least 10 of which aid the phenomenon known as autofluorescence by serving as fluorophores.
- There are other autofluorescence phenomena in the ocular fundus; autofluorescence in the lipofuscin can basically be traced back to RPE in vivo.
- Measurement of fundus autofluorescence (FAF) is a noninvasive procedure that uses the lipofuscin accumulation as a parameter for assessing the RPE in various diseases.

Procedure

- FAF measurements are usually carried out with confocal scanning laser ophthalmoscopes such as the Heidelberg Retina Angiograph (HRA; Heidelberg Engineering, Heidelberg, Germany).
- Excitation takes place with an argon blue laser (488 nm) and is measured by appropriate filtering of the emitted light only above 500 nm.
- A series of up to 30 consecutive images are taken. To optimize the signal-to-noise ratio, selected images are digitally aligned. This allows examination even in small children or less cooperative patients, in whom a few optimal images can be selected from a larger photographic series.
- In cooperative patients, FAF can be measured with undilated pupils with the HRA.
- FAF can be measured with fundus cameras, but the images appear to be different due to a broader range of excitation wavelengths in contrast with laser excitation, different filtering, or the nonconfocal observation mode.

Normal Fundus Autofluorescence

- The retinal vessels lie as dark shadows in front of the autofluorescence of the RPE. The optic disc is also dark.
- A decrease in the autofluorescence is evident in the fovea, resulting from a blockage from the yellow macular pigment and a lower amount of lipofuscin in the pigment epithelium cells under the fovea. The size of this central decrease in the fluorescence is variable between normal individuals.
- The strongest autofluorescence exists in a ring on the edge of the macula. Further into the periphery, the lipofuscin content of the RPE cells and the autofluorescence decreases.
- The diagnostic method allows evaluation of the divergence of the autofluorescence distribution from the normal patterns and of individual changes in the course of the disease.
- Interindividual comparisons are difficult due to the variable optical media and the variable laser intensities used.

Pathological Findings

- Increased autofluorescence corresponds to increased lipofuscin content and consequently a possible degenerative process. In some circumstances, increased autofluorescence can also be caused by the displacement of pigment epithelial cells in choroidal processes.
- Reduced autofluorescence can relate to reduced development of lipofuscin, a lack of pigment epithelium cells, or blockage by vessels, blood, or other causes.
- Changes in autofluorescence reflect pathological processes, but do not correlate directly with retinal function. For example, an increased ring of autofluorescence indicates the border of a functioning central retina in retinitis pigmentosa, and the area of most severe functional loss in chloroquine retinopathy.

Clinical Applications

- Numerous retinal diseases have been investigated in small series using FAF. However, there is still a need for larger series with long-term follow-up to confirm the diagnostic and prognostic relevance of the method.
- The major advantage of the method is early detection of morphological abnormalities when ophthalmoscopy is still normal.
- In principle, FAF can replace invasive fluorescein angiography in all nonexudative retinal diseases. It is also simpler to apply when monitoring the course of a disease.
- In age-related maculopathy, patterns of early disease development have recently been established.
- In age-related macular degeneration, it has been demonstrated that areas of increased autofluorescence at the edge of geographic atrophy mark the areas that will next be affected by the atrophy.
- In hereditary retinal dystrophies, alterations in the RPE become visible that are not evident on ophthalmoscopy or fluorescein angiography. Areas of increased autofluorescence—e. g., in retinitis pigmentosa—indicate the border of functioning retina.
- In chloroquine retinal toxicity, increased autofluorescence can become visible before abnormalities on ophthalmoscopy or fluorescein angiography.
- Exudative changes become visible with increased autofluorescence, and their regression can be observed using autofluorescence.

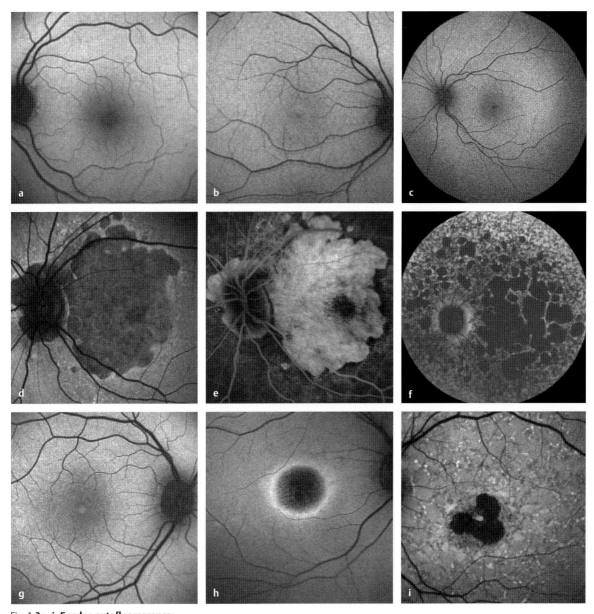

Fig. 1.3a–i Fundus autofluorescence

a Fundus autofluorescence. A normal distribution of autofluorescence.

b Fundus autofluorescence (different patient). A normal distribution of autofluorescence. It should be noted that the central area of reduced autofluorescence is different in comparison with **a**.

c Fundus autofluorescence (different patient). Wide-angle imaging with normal distribution of autofluorescence.

d Fundus autofluorescence. Retinochoroidal dystrophy at the posterior pole in a young woman. Areas of pigment epithelial loss show reduced autofluorescence. The border zone shows increased fluorescence, probably corresponding to areas of progressive degeneration.

e Fluorescein angiography (same patient as in **d**). In the late phase, the loss of the choriocapillaris and retinal pigment epithelium is indicated by hyperfluorescence without leakage. The area corresponds to the lesion depicted in fundus autofluorescence.

f Fundus autofluorescence (different patient). A wide-angle image of severe cone–rod dystrophy, with confluent patchy loss of retinal pigment epithelium.

g Fundus autofluorescence. Foveal dystrophy, with increased foveal autofluorescence as the only morphological pathological finding when ophthalmoscopy was normal.

h Fundus autofluorescence. Macular dystrophy, with central loss of autofluorescence and a ring of increased autofluorescence.

i Fundus autofluorescence. Stargardt disease, with central retinal pigment epithelium atrophy and multiple flecks (fundus flavimaculatus).

- Imaging of drusen in the optic disc is facilitated.
- Differentiation between choroidal melanoma and choroidal nevi may be facilitated by different patterns in autofluorescence in small melanocytic uveal lesions.

References

Bellmann C, Rubin GS, Kabanarou SA, et al. Fundus autofluorescence imaging compared with different confocal ophthalmoscopes. Br J Ophthalmol 2003;87:1381–6.

Bindewald A, Bird AC, Dandekar SS. Classification of fundus autofluorescence patterns in early age-related macular disease. Invest Ophthalmol Vis Sci 2005;46:3309–14.

Bindewald A, Schmitz-Valckenberg S, Jorzik JJ, et al. Classification of abnormal fundus autofluorescence patterns in the junctional zone of geographic atrophy in patients with age-related macular degeneration. Br J Ophthalmol 2005;89:874–8.

Delori FC, Dorey CK, Staurenghi G, Arend O, Goger DG, Weiter JJ. In vivo fluorescence of the ocular fundus exhibits retinal pigment epithelium lipofuscin characteristics. Invest Ophthalmol Vis Sci 1995;36:718–29.

Eldred GE. Age pigment structure. Nature 1993;364:396.

Robson AG, Egan CA, Luong VA, et al. Comparison of fundus autofluorescence with photopic and scotopic fine-matrix mapping in patients with retinitis pigmentosa and normal visual acuity. Invest Ophthalomol Vis Sci 2004;45:4119–25.

Spaide RF, Klancnik JM Jr. Fundus autofluorescence and central serous chorioretinopathy. Ophthalmology 2005;112:825–33.

Wabbels B, Demmler A, Paunescu K, Wegscheider E, Preising MN, Lorenz B. Fundus autofluorescence in children and teenagers with hereditary retinal diseases. Graefes Arch Clin Exp Ophthalmol 2006;244:36–45.

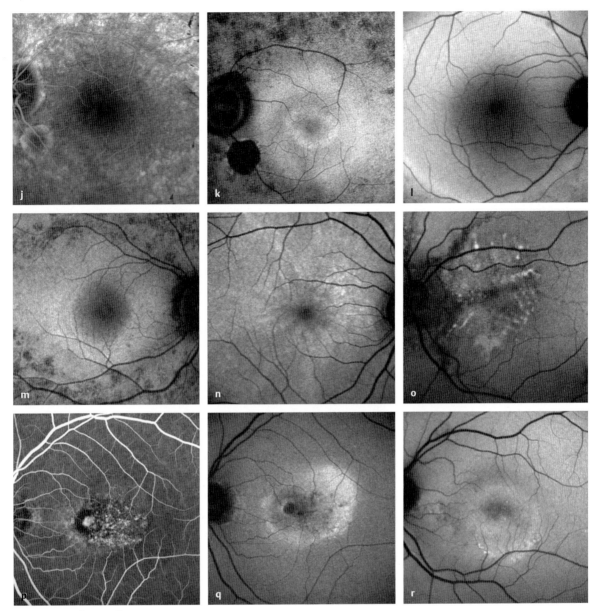

Fig. 1.3j–r Fundus autofluorescence

j Fluorescein angiography. Retinitis pigmentosa with peripheral choriocapillaris atrophy and a chorioretinal atrophic lesion below the optic disc (see section 4.1).

k Fundus autofluorescence (same patient as in **j**). The areas of retinal pigment epithelium loss are more clearly outlined with fundus autofluorescence in comparison with fluorescein angiography. In addition, the pericentral ring of increased autofluorescence is not detectable with ophthalmoscopy or fluorescein angiography.

l Fundus autofluorescence. Retinitis pigmentosa, with a large ring of increased autofluorescence at the vascular arcades.

m Fundus autofluorescence. Retinitis pigmentosa, with a smaller ring of increased autofluorescence at the posterior pole and patchy loss of autofluorescence toward the periphery.

n Fundus autofluorescence. Irregularities on fundus autofluorescence in a carrier of X-linked retinitis pigmentosa.

o Fundus autofluorescence. Angioid streaks are visible as dark lines originating from the disk. Although no exudative activity was detected on angiography, flecks of increased autofluorescence indicate active metabolic processes (see section 8.6).

p Fluorescein angiography. A small choroidal neovascularization.

q Fundus autofluorescence (same patient as in **p**). The area of the accompanying exudation is indicated by increased autofluorescence. Autofluorescence is blocked in the area of the neovascularization.

r Fundus autofluorescence (different patient). Increased autofluorescence indicates the area of exudation in central serous chorioretinopathy (see section 8.1).

1.4 Stereo Angiography *Werner Inhoffen*

Basic Principle

- Spatial definition of the phenomena made visible by fluorescein angiography is often difficult or impossible—for example, leakages from the retinal tissue are difficult to differentiate from those of choroidal origin. It is also impossible, for example, to detect slightly elevated pigment epithelium—e. g., in occult choroidal neovascularization (CNV).
- However, a useful three-dimensional image can be obtained with two single images derived from two different angles of observation. This technique, in which paired images are evaluated using special technology, is known as stereo angiography.

Advantages of Stereo Angiography

- Identification of elevated structures of the choroid or the retinal pigment epithelium (RPE): CNV, pigment epithelial detachment (PED), and identification of choroidal tumors.
- Identification of elevated retinal structures (e. g., in macular edema, neurosensory detachment).
- Differentiation of hyperfluorescent structures inside the retinal layer (e. g., microaneurysms) and around the RPE layer (e. g., leakages in central serous chorioretinopathy).

Procedure

- The following techniques are possible:
  - Angiography with a special camera (the full stereo technique, with a fixed recording angle in which both exposures are taken simultaneously).
  - The technique most often used involves a standard fundus camera and taking two images subsequently (a pseudostereo technique), using lateral movement (most frequently) or vertical movement of the camera head (less common).
- Pseudostereo technique with lateral movement. To obtain images with sufficient stereo effect, a slight displacement of the camera to the left and then to the right should be carried out while ensuring that the unilluminated central observation area of the camera remains on the patient's pupil. The displacements have to be made very quickly to avoid eye movements by the patient and to guarantee comparable filling patterns in the early phase in both images.
- Application. Stereo angiography can be applied not only in ophthalmoscopy, but is also practical for fluorescein angiography and indocyanine green angiography, and

can be carried out using a digital or a conventional fundus camera and also with laser scanning equipment (e. g., the Heidelberg Retina Angiograph scanning laser ophthalmoscope, Heidelberg Engineering, Germany).

Evaluation of Stereo Angiography

- Paper print-out as a stereo pair (with the left image next to the right image). The centers of both images should not lie further than 6 cm from each other. When examining the images using lenses of +3 D up to +5 D, one should move in close to the pair of images and slowly increase the distance of the head from the images until a new three-dimensional image appears located between the two original images.
- Paper print-out as an anaglyph. This is a single image in which the two images are superimposed (with slight lateral displacement) and colored differently (red or green). To separate them visually, the images have to be viewed with red–green (three-dimensional) spectacles.
- As a negative image. A stereo pair on a light box can be viewed using a stereo viewer (e. g., Topcon, Japan).
- In an auditorium, using two slide projectors with polarization filters in front of the focusing lenses, with the difference in the polarization angles of the left and right projector filters amounting to 90°. The two images are projected on top of each other onto a special screen; viewers wear polarized spectacles to see them.
- On the computer screen. The pair of images can be observed with prisms, mirror systems, or with shutter spectacles (the accessories are available from fundus camera system providers).

References

Frambach DA, Dacey MP, Sadun A. Stereoscopic photography with a scanning laser ophthalmoscope. Am J Ophthalmol 1993;116: 484–8.

Gass JD. Diseases causing choroidal exudative and hemorrhagic localized (disciform) detachment of the retina and retinal pigment epithelium, In: Gass JD, ed. Stereoscopic atlas of macular diseases: diagnosis and treatment, 4th ed. St. Louis: Mosby, 1997:49–285.

Orlock D. Special techniques using the conventional ICG fundus camera: digital stereo imaging. In: Flower LA, Slakter RW, Yannuzzi L, eds. Indocyanine green angiography. London: Mosby, 1997: 63–71.

Sandhu SS, Talks SJ. Correlation of optical coherence tomography, with or without additional color fundus photography, with stereo fundus fluorescein angiography in diagnosing choroidal neovascular membranes. Br J Ophthalmol 2005;89:967–70.

Tyler ME. Stereo fundus photography: principle and technique. In: Tyler ME, Saine PJ, eds. Ophthalmic photography. Oxford: Butterworth-Heinemann, 1997: 79–116 (2nd ed. 2002).

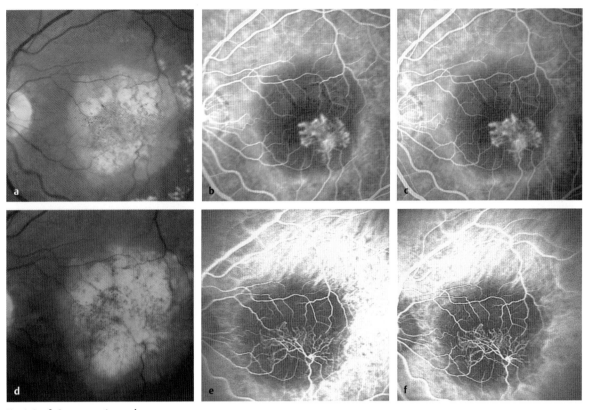

Fig. 1.4a–f Stereo angiography

a Color photograph. Patient with a pigment epithelium detachment (a more or less yellow circular area), with isolated areas of atrophy resulting from resorption of drusen.

b Early arteriovenous phase. Digital fluorescein angiography in the left-hand position. The pigment epithelium detachment appears dark here and therefore contrasts well with the visible vessels of the choroidal neovascularization.

c Early arteriovenous phase, shortly after image **b** was taken, and with the camera in the right-hand position. Looking at **b** and **c** simultaneously, a stereo image appears with a choroidal neovascularization arising from the anastomosis area, just beneath the retina in the area of pigment epithelium detachment. The surface configuration of the pigment epithelium detachment is also clearly visible.

d Color photograph. The same patient 7 months later, with no essential changes in the diagnostic findings in the fundus.

e High-speed indocyanine green angiography with the HRA camera in the left-hand position. The pigment epithelium detachment also appears dark here, and so contrasts well with the vessels of the subretinal neovascularization. The vessels in the choroidal neovascularization are clearly recognizable and have grown along the surface of the pigment epithelium detachment.

f High speed indocyanine green angiography 1 s later, in the right-hand position. When **e** and **f** are examined simultaneously, the resulting spatial image shows the afferent retinal vessels from the lower edge of the pigment epithelium detachment more clearly than in a nonstereo image and also more clearly than in a fluorescein image. The chorioretinal anastomosis is probably part of a retinal angiomatous proliferation. In contrast, the pigment epithelium detachment in the fluorescein angiogram is easier to recognize, as more structures covering its surface are visible.

1.5 Comparison of Retinal Imaging Methods   *Ulrich Kellner*

History of Retinal Imaging

- For decades, ophthalmoscopy, fundus photography, fluorescein angiography, and diagnostic ultrasound were the only methods of retinal imaging. In the last 20 years, several techniques have been developed: indocyanine angiography, optical coherence tomography, scanning laser ophthalmoscopy (SLO), fundus autofluorescence, infrared imaging, and macular pigment density measurements. Additional developments include digital technology, which allows easy processing and storage of data as well as easy worldwide exchange of images and wide-angle lenses. Today, the retinal specialist is able to choose from a range of imaging methods, with the prospect of future developments in various areas for even more detailed retinal examination.

Fundus Photography

- Fundus photography rarely makes it possible to detect more abnormalities than with ophthalmoscopy, but the advantage of the method is that it allows documentation of retinal abnormalities either for detailed analysis (e. g., drusen counting), comparison with other imaging methods or with the findings during follow-up examinations, and easy exchange between examiners with digital photography to improve the quality of diagnosis—e. g., with telemedicine.

Infrared Reflectance

- Spectral imaging has been available for decades, but the requirement for special film and illumination equipment prevented it from coming into widespread use. Infrared imaging with a confocal scanning laser ophthalmoscope (HRA, Heidelberg Engineering Ltd., Heidelberg, Germany) makes it possible to detect epiretinal membranes and abnormalities in the pigment epithelium.
- Infrared imaging may make it easier to identify retinal abnormalities that are difficult to detect with ophthalmoscopy and that may be in contrast to the results of other imaging techniques. The diagnostic yield of infrared imaging is as yet undetermined, but it is easy to document before fundus autofluorescence or fluorescein angiography.

Fundus Autofluorescence

- Research in the field of fundus autofluorescence (FAF) imaging using the HRA has recently shown the advantages of this easy and noninvasive imaging technique for nonexudative fundus lesions. FAF reflects the metabolic state of the retinal pigment epithelium (RPE) and, in addition to demonstrating RPE abnormalities, makes it possible to visualize areas with active degenerative processes. FAF can therefore provide additional information in comparison with fluorescein angiography. In some cases, FAF may be the only method of detecting morphological abnormalities (e. g., macular dystrophy, chloroquine retinopathy), facilitating earlier diagnosis of retinal disorders.
- FAF can be recommended as the first choice for fundus imaging instead of fluorescein angiography in nonexudative fundus lesions. Additional advantages include easy follow-up and the ability to examine even small children. In addition, FAF can also be used for description and follow-up in exudative fundus lesions.

Wide-Angle Fundus Imaging

- Most retinal disorders that require detailed imaging for diagnosis affect the posterior pole. However, in some disorders, wide-angle imaging is of value—e. g., in conditions affecting the periphery (diabetic retinopathy, screening for retinopathy of prematurity, peripheral tumors). Wide-angle imaging is possible with fundus camera systems (e. g., Carl Zeiss Meditec, Inc., Jena, Germany; Topcon Corporation, Tokyo, Japan), confocal scanning laser ophthalmoscopes (HRA) or wide-angle scanning laser ophthalmoscopes (Panoramic 200, Optos, United Kingdom). Wide-angle imaging involves a loss of detail, but a complete fundus overview can be of major importance, particularly in telemedicine.
- The RetCam (Clarity Medical Systems, Pleasanton, CA, USA) is a wide-angle digital pediatric retinal imaging system that is used to document retinopathy of prematurity or retinoblastomas.

Fluorescein and Indocyanine Green Angiography

- The major advantage of these two angiographic methods is that they make it possible to visualize dynamic processes in the retinal and choroidal vascular network, as well as fluid exchanges between different compartments in the retina or choroid. The continuous development of hyperfluorescent leakage in the course of the angiogram cannot be observed with any other imaging method.
- The recent development of less invasive imaging methods has changed the indications in two major respects. In nonexudative lesions, fundus autofluorescence should replace angiography as the method of choice whenever it is available. In exudative lesions, the development of the lesion after treatment can also be observed with optical coherence tomography or other methods of measuring the retinal thickness, reducing the need for repeated angiographies to assess the course of the disease.
- Fluorescein angiography is still the method of choice for diagnosis in all vascular and exudative retinal or choroidal disorders. Indocyanine angiography has a limited impact on the diagnosis of macular disorders and should be used to differentiate certain retinal and choroidal diseases.

Macular Pigment Density Measurements

- Interest in the relevance of macular pigment for macular degenerations resulted in the development of several techniques for measuring the density of the macular pigment (such as Raman spectroscopy, heterochromatic flicker photometry, two-wavelength autofluorescence with a modified confocal scanning laser ophthalmoscope, two-wavelength reflectance imaging). All of these techniques have advantages and disadvantages and are still undergoing further development. It has been shown that the density and distribution of the macular pigment varies among healthy individuals. Similarly, the effect of lutein intake is variable in different individuals. A clear effect of macular pigment density on macular degeneration has not yet been demonstrated. The clinical value of macular pigment density measurements will depend on future research on the role of macular pigment in retinal disease.

Optical Coherence Tomography

- The advantage of optical coherence tomography (OCT; Carl Zeiss Meditec, Inc., Jena, Germany) is that it allows detailed analysis of retinal structures similar to that provided by histological images. Documentation of epiretinal membranes, macular holes, the stages of macular hole healing after surgery, macular edema, subretinal fluid, choroidal neovascularization before and after treatment, and abnormalities of the optic disc are only some of the applications for this technique. Particularly in follow-up examinations after the treatment of exudative macular disorders, OCT is capable of replacing fluorescein angiography. In addition, macular edema can be detected before it becomes clinically evident.
- The major disadvantage of the current technology is its dependence on the position of the individual scans and their overlap. Promising future developments include higher resolution and off-line slicing of a complete three-dimensional scan of the posterior pole.

Retinal Thickness Analysis

- Different methods are available for measuring retinal thickness—e. g., in diabetic macular edema: optical coherence tomography (OCT); the Retinal Thickness Analyzer (RTA, Talia Technology Ltd., Lod, Israel) and the macular module of the Heidelberg Retina Tomograph (HRT, Heidelberg Engineering Ltd., Heidelberg, Germany). Recent studies have shown that it is possible to measure the retinal thickness with all of these methods, but that the methods are poorly comparable. To date, none of these techniques has shown any clear advantages in relation to the analysis of retinal thickness. Other imaging facilities differ between the instruments and may therefore influence the choice of an individual technique.

Combination Techniques

- Recently, a combination of OCT and the scanning laser ophthalmoscope (OCT Ophthalmoscope, Ophthalmic Technologies, Inc., Toronto, Ontario, Canada) has been developed. Experience with this technique is as yet limited.

Retinal Vessel Analysis

- Different techniques have been used to measure retinal vessel diameters on fundus images. Presently, the diagnostic impact of retinal vessel analysis regarding ocular and extraocular vascular disease is under discussion. Future research is focused on functional data that are obtained when measuring the dilation of retinal vessels under flicker stimulation (Dynamic Vessel Analyzer, IMEDOS, Jena, Germany) or slow multifocal stimulation.

Retinal Imaging for Glaucoma

- Imaging of the optic disc and the retinal nerve fiber layer has become standard for glaucoma in research and clinical practice. Imaging techniques developed for glaucoma research (HRT) have been used for macular imaging and vice versa (OCT, RTA). In addition, scanning laser polarimetry can be used for nerve fiber analysis (GDx VCC, Carl Zeiss Meditec, Inc., Jena, Germany). Currently, most data are available for the HRT. A limited number of comparative studies with two or three instruments have been reported, indicating that each technique is reliable. Comparison between different instruments, however, is limited and the same technique should be used for follow-up in a single patient.

Diagnostic Ultrasonography

- Diagnostic ultrasound is an important method for evaluating the integrity of the retina, particularly in opacified ocular media, for documenting and measuring intraocular tumors, and for evaluating orbital abnormalities. With regard to retinal imaging, the resolution of this technique is limited, and optical coherence tomography provides much more detail in comparison with ultrasonography. One advantage is the use of ultrasound biomicroscopy in the anterior segments of the retina, especially for diagnosing tumors, in a region that is inaccessible for all other imaging methods. The advantage of diagnostic ultrasound is its easy use and widespread availability; the major disadvantage is still its dependence on the individual examiner.

References

Davies NP, Morland AB. Macular pigments: their characteristics and putative role. Prog Retin Eye Res 2004;23:533–59.

Hoffmann EM, Bowd C, Medeiros FA, et al: Agreement among 3 optical imaging methods for the assessment of optic disc topography. Ophthalmology 2005;112:2149–56

Goebel W, Franke R: Retinal thickness in diabetic retinopathy: comparison of optic coherence tomography, the retinal thickness analyzer, and fundus photography. Retina 2006;26:49–57

Montero JA, Ruiz-Moreno JM. Macular thickness in patients with choroidal neovascularization determined by RTA and OCT3: comparative results. Eye 2005;19:72–6.

Schmidt-Erfurth U, Leitgeb RA, Michels S, et al. Three-dimensional ultrahigh resolution optical coherence tomography of macular diseases. Invest Ophthalmol Vis Sci 2005;46:3393–402

Yanuzzi LA, Ober MD, Slakter JS, et al. Ophthalmic fundus imaging: today and beyond. Am J Ophthalmol 2004;137:511–24.

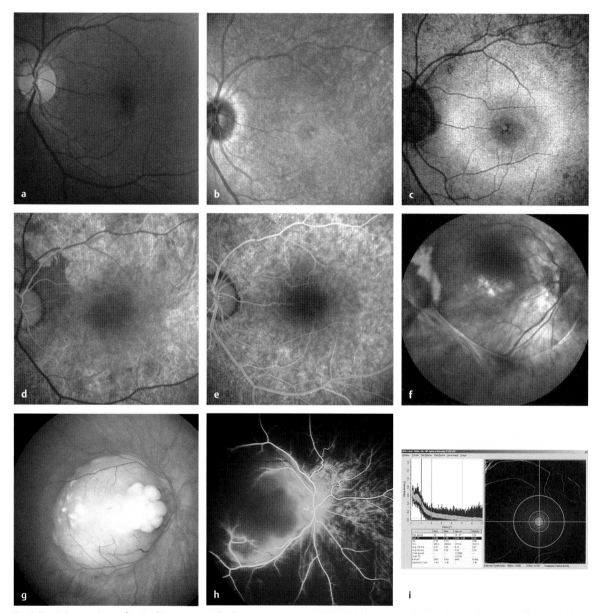

Fig. 1.5a–i Comparison of retinal imaging methods

a Color photograph: 44-year old patient with autosomal dominant retinitis pigmentosa. The color photography shows narrowed vessels, otherwise the retina at the posterior pole appears not to be severely altered.

b Infrared imaging: In addition to the color photograph, the retinal pigment epithelium (RPE) appears to have multiple small fleck-like irregularities

c Fundus autofluorescence (FAF): Foveal irregular distribution of FAF is surrounded by a ring of increased FAF, beyond the vascular arcades patchy loss of FAF indicates patchy loss of RPE.

d Fluorescein angiography, early phase: Loss of RPE is indicated by the good visibility of large choroidal vessels.

e Late phase: The fovea appears normal without cystoid macular edema, whereas towards the periphery increased choroidal fluorescence indicates loss of RPE.

f Wide-field infrared imaging (different patient): Vitreoretinal tractional membranes are present in this patient with retinitis pigmentosa and temporal Coats-like vascular alterations.

g Wide-field imaging in infants (RetCam): A retinoblastoma affects the posterior pole (courtesy of A. Schueler, Bremen, Germany).

h Wide-field fluorescein angiography (RetCam): In the early phase the retinoblastoma shows blockage. This image was taken in a study to identify possible fluorescein angiographic characteristics of treated retinoblastoma. Fluorescein angiography is not recommended for diagnosis of retinoblastoma (courtesy of A. Schueler, Bremen, Germany).

i Macular pigment measurement: In the image on the right the difference between two FAF images at different wavelengths is used to calculate macular pigment density (MPD). The density peaks in the fovea indicated by the bright spot. The left image displays the radial distribution of MPD. Different patterns of radial distribution have been described (courtesy of S. Wolf, Bern, Switzerland)

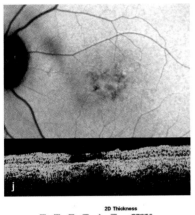

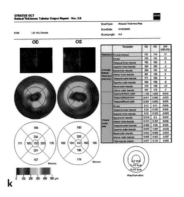

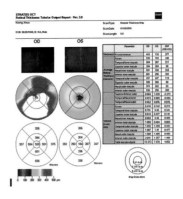

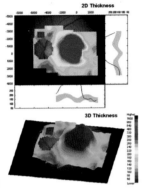

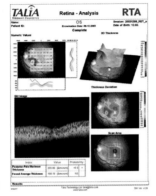

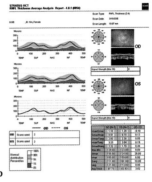

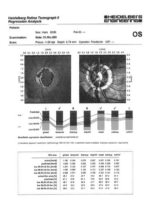

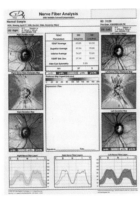

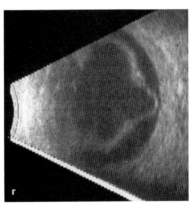

Fig. 1.5j–r Comparison of retinal imaging methods

j FAF and Optic Coherence Tomography (OCT) in a patient with cone-rod dystrophy: FAF irregularities are displayed in the fovea (upper image). The diagonal line on the left is due to vitreous floaters. The OCT (lower image) indicates loss of retinal thickness and cystoid lesions in the fovea.

k OCT retinal thickness map (same patient as **j**): The blue colors indicate loss of retinal thickness at the posterior pole in both eyes.

l OCT retinal thickness map (different patient): In a patient with diabetic retinopathy, diabetic macular edema is present in the right eye (indicated by red and white areas), whereas retinal thickness is normal on the left eye (indicated by green and yellow colors).

m Retinal Thickness Analyzer (RTA) imaging: 2D and 3D retinal thickness distribution in a different patient with diabetic macular edema. The red colors indicate increased retinal thickness (courtesy of A.S. Neubauer, Munich, Germany).

n RTA imaging report in a patient with paracentral serous chorioretinopathy: A circumscribed increase of retinal thickness is indicated by red colors in the lower nasal macular area (courtesy of A.S. Neubauer, Munich, Germany).

o OCT: Retinal nerve fiber layer measurement report in a normal proband.

p Optic disc tomography (Heidelberg Retina Tomograph) in a patient with progressed glaucomatous damage on the left eye.

q Retinal Nerve Fiber Analysis with a GDx VCC in a patient with normal left eye and suspected glaucoma on the right eye (courtesy of Carl Zeiss Meditec AG, Jena, Germany).

r Ultrasonography: Good overview of a longstanding retinal detachment with increased retinal thickness and proliferative vitreoretinopathy.

2 Adverse Effects of Fluorescein and Indocyanine Green Angiography *Jan Breckwoldt and Ulrich Kellner*

Adverse Effects of Fluorescein Angiography

- Intravenously injected sodium fluorescein is generally tolerated without any major problems. Possible side effects can be classified as mild (approximately one in 20 to one in 100 angiographies), moderate (approximately one in 60), and serious (approximately one in 2000).
- Fatalities have been reported in at least seven cases immediately after fluorescein angiography, and a frequency of one in 220 000 has been calculated.
- The incidence of adverse effects appears to have decreased in recent years due to the availability of better fluorescein preparations.
- In practice, the most common side effect observed is nausea some 30 s after injection. This is generally self-limiting, but it often coincides with the important phase of arteriovenous transfer and, because of resultant restricted photographic conditions, can seriously reduce the quality of the angiography.
- However, despite the rarity of serious side effects, the physician supervising an angiography must be able to recognize serious emergencies and provide appropriate treatment.
- Oral administration of fluorescein has been suggested as an alternative method; however, an anaphylactic reaction after oral administration has also been observed.

Adverse Effects of Indocyanine Green Angiography

- Intravenously injected indocyanine green (ICG) is generally tolerated without any major problems. Adverse effects can be classified as mild (0.15–0.26% of ICG angiographies), moderate (0.2% of ICG angiographies), or serious (0.05% of ICG angiographies).
- Nausea is less frequent than with fluorescein angiography.
- Anaphylactic shock has been reported in some patients.
- As indocyanine green preparations may contain iodine, care should be taken in patients who are known to have allergic reactions to iodine and in patients with thyroid disease.

Possible Mechanisms of Adverse Effects

- Vasovagal reaction (bradycardia, hypotension, reduced cardiac perfusion).
- Allergic reaction (with evidence of IgE, IgG4, or complement activation).
- Nonallergic histamine release (anaphylactoid reaction).
- Anxiety-based sympathetic activation (possibly with tachycardic myocardial ischemia).
- Vasospastic effects of the substance.
- Effects due to contamination of the applied substance.
- Systemic effects of topical mydriatics.
- Any combination of the above.

Anaphylactic Shock

- Anaphylactic shock is a rare adverse effect of fluorescein or indocyanine green angiography that can quickly develop into a life-threatening situation. The incidence is approximately one in 2000 examinations.
- Anaphylactic and anaphylactoid reactions do not differ either in their clinical profiles or the respective acute treatments.
- From the methodological point of view, the severity of an anaphylactic reaction should be classified according to clinical stages; different organ systems can develop completely different stages side by side.
- Therapeutic action should be adequate to tackle the developing threat to the patient. In some cases, rapid and specific intervention is essential. Because of the rarity of these cases, it is important for the medical team to have regular training sessions to familiarize themselves with procedures and equipment. Training should take place at the home institution and should reflect realistic situations as accurately as possible.
- Clinical phenomena are prompted by vasodilation, capillary leakage, and cell edema, leading to the clinical phenomena listed in Table 2.1.

Table 2.1 Clinical effects of vasodilation, capillary leakage and cellular edema

Cardiovascular system	Intravascular volume depletion, tachycardia, reduction of the cardiac oxygen reserve
Respiratory tract	Laryngeal edema, bronchospasm
Gastrointestinal, mucosal, and cutaneous signs	Abdominal pain, nausea, vomiting, urticaria, rhinitis, erythema or paleness

Clinical Stages and Therapy

Table 2.**2** Clinical staging and treatment

Stage	I	II	III	IV
Clinical signs	Disseminated cutaneous reactions, mucosal edema, nonspecific symptoms	Tachycardia, falling blood pressure, dyspnea, urge to urinate and defecate	Manifest hemodynamic shock, severe bronchospasm, loss of consciousness	Cardiocirculatory arrest

Therapy	I. v. H_1 and H_2 blockers:
	– Clemastine 2 mg
	– Cimetidine 300 mg
		In addition: i. v. volume
		– Crystalloids (containing isotonic saline)
		– Adrenergic agents/bronchodilators: Epinephrine i. m. or s. c. (0.3–0.5 mg) or inhaled (0.1 mg/ml)
			In addition:
			– Colloids (hetastarch)
			– Vasopressors
			  • Epinephrine i. v. (starting with 0.1 mg/ min titrated to clinical signs; if appropriate > 1 mg)
			  • Norepinephrine i. v. (dosage as epinephrine)
				In addition: Cardiopulmonary resuscitation (CPR)
				– Start CPR if no sign of circulation for 10 s
				– Cardiac massage and rescue breathing (ratio 30 : 2), frequency of chest compressions 100/min

	I. v. corticosteroids – Prednisolone 50–125 mg	I. v. corticosteroids – Prednisolone 250–500 mg	I. v. corticosteroids – Prednisolone 1000 mg	

I. m.: intramuscular; i. v.: intravenous; s. c.: subcutaneous.

References

Bonte CA, Ceuppens J, Leys AM. Hypotensive shock as a complication of infracyanine green injection. Retina 1998;18:476–7.

Chamberlain D. Emergency medical treatment of anaphylactic reactions. Project Team of the Resuscitation Council (UK). J Accid Emerg Med 1999;16:243–7.

Gomez-Ulla F, Gutierrez C, Seoane I. Severe anaphylactic reaction to orally administered fluorescein. Am J Ophthalmol 1991;112:94.

Hitosugi M, Omura K, Yokoyama T, et al. An autopsy case of fatal anaphylactic shock following fluorescein angiography: a case report. Med Sci Law 2004;44:264–5.

Jennings BJ, Mathews DE. Adverse reactions during retinal fluorescein angiography. J Am Optom Assoc 1994;65:465–71.

Obana A, Miki T, Hayashi K, et al. Survey of complications of indocyanine green angiography in Japan. Am J Ophthalmol 1994;118:749–53.

Olsen TW, Lim JI, Capone A Jr, Myles RA, Gilman JP. Anaphylactic shock following indocyanine green angiography. Arch Ophthalmol 1996;114:97

Soar J, Deakin CD, Nolan JP, et al. European Resuscitation Council Guideline for Resuscitation 2005. Section 7g: Anaphylaxis. Resuscitation 2005;67S1:151–5

Yannuzzi LA, Rohrer KT, Tindel LJ, et al. Fluorescein angiography complication survey. Ophthalmology 1986;93:611–7.

3.1 Classification of Age-Related Macular Disease   *Joachim Wachtlin*

Definitions and Classification

- Different terms are used to identify subgroups of patients with age-related macular disease.
- Age-related macular disease can be subdivided into early and late stages. The early stages present with development of drusen and hyperpigmentation or hypopigmentation of the retinal pigment epithelium. Late stages with severe visual loss include the development of choroidal neovascularization (CNV), pigment epithelial detachment, subretinal hemorrhage, or geographic atrophy.
- The early stages have been termed age-related maculopathy (ARM) in contrast to the late stages, which are known as age-related macular degeneration (AMD or ARMD). The acronyms AMD and ARMD are used for both age-related macular disease and for age-related macular degeneration.
- The late stages have also often been subdivided into a nonexudative or "dry" form, corresponding to geographic atrophy, and an exudative or "wet" form, including CNV, pigment epithelial detachment, and associated subretinal hemorrhage.
- Drusen as a major indicator of age-related macular disease have been subdivided into well-defined "hard" drusen and less distinct "soft" drusen, which are distinguished by size.
- CNVs are differentiated into classic or occult, on the basis of the fluorescein-angiographic findings in the early phases of the angiogram.

Epidemiology, Pathophysiology, and Clinical Presentation

- Age-related macular disease is the most prevalent form of macular disease in the elderly and is the leading cause of blindness in people over the age of 50 in industrialized countries.
- The incidence and prevalence of different stages of age-related macular disease have been established in large population-based studies conducted in the USA, the Netherlands, and Australia.
- In large epidemiological studies, the prevalence of age-related macular degeneration is reported to range from approximately 0.2% in patients aged 55–64 up to 11% in those over 85. Age-related maculopathy is 4–10 times more common, depending on age.
- Visual loss develops in the late stages in approximately 85% of nonexudative lesions and 15% of exudative lesions.
- Risk factors consistently found in these studies are increasing age, a positive family history, and smoking—the latter being the only risk factor capable of being influenced. The potential influence of other factors such as nutrition or cataract surgery is a matter of debate.
- Genetic predisposition has been suspected on the basis of family and twin studies. Recently, polymorphisms in the CHF gene and the LOC387715 gene have been identified that are associated with an increased risk of age-related macular disease.

- The pathophysiology has not yet been completely clarified. A multifactorial process influenced by aging leads to dysfunction of the functional complex of photoreceptors, retinal pigment epithelium, and Bruch membrane.
- The classic symptoms are deterioration in visual acuity and metamorphopsia.
- The process leads to an extensive central scotoma and the development of paracentral fixation. Reading and recognition of faces are no longer possible.
- If only one eye is affected, the healthy eye will compensate for the deficiency in the diseased eye, so that the condition in the affected eye is often only discovered incidentally.
- The decline of visual function takes place significantly more quickly in exudative age-related macular degeneration than in the nonexudative form.
- Peripheral vision is usually preserved, and spatial orientation is also possible in the late phases of the disease.
- About 30% of patients with advanced AMD suffer depression, an aspect that is commonly underestimated.

Diagnosis and Treatment

- The diagnosis is established by ophthalmoscopy. Fluorescein angiography makes it possible to differentiate most forms of age-related macular disease and is mandatory for many treatment decisions. Fundus autofluorescence, optical coherence tomography, and indocyanine angiography provide additional information for subclassifying the disease, taking decisions regarding treatment, and establishing the follow-up procedures required.
- Amsler grid tests can be used for self-screening.
- Treatment options are stage-dependent and include substitution of nutrients, laser coagulation, photodynamic therapy, macular surgery, intravitreal injection of drugs, and low-vision aids.
- Affected patients and family members at risk should be advised to stop smoking.

References

Bird AC. Age-related macular disease. Br J Ophthalmol 1996;80:1–2.

Bird AC, Bressler NM, Bressler SB, et al. An international classification and grading system for age-related maculopathy and age-related macular degeneration. The International ARM Epidemiological Study Group. Surv Ophthalmol 1995;39:367–74.

Haines JL, Hauser MA, Schmidt S, et al. Complement factor H variant increases the risk of age-related macular degeneration. Science 2005;308:419–21.

Klein R, Peto T, Bird A, Vannekirk MR. The epidemiology of age-related macular disease. Am J Ophthalmol 2004;137:486–95.

Rivera A, Fisher SA, Fritsche LG, et al. Hypothetical LOC387715 is a second major susceptibility gene for age-related macular degeneration, contributing independently of complement factor H to disease risk. Hum Mol Genet 2005;14:3227–36.

Thornton J, Edwards R, Mitchell P, et al. Smoking and age-related macular degeneration: a review of association. Eye 2005;19:935–44.

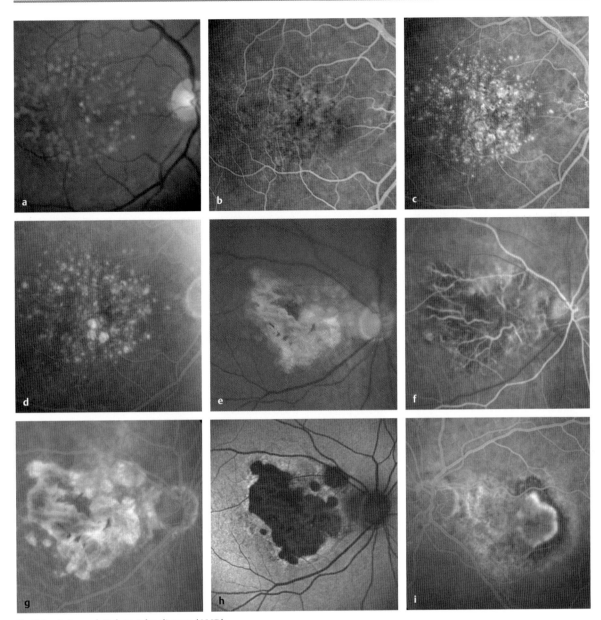

Fig. 3.1a–i Age-related macular disease (AMD)

a Color photograph. Age-related maculopathy, with soft and hard drusen presenting as yellow–white subretinal deposits.

b Early phase. Temporal to the fovea, the hard drusen can be distinguished as small, well-defined, hyperfluorescent lesions.

c Late arteriovenous phase. The hard drusen have reached maximum hyperfluorescence and are clearly distinguishable. The soft drusen have become more visible, with less distinct borders.

d Late phase. Hyperfluorescence in the area of the soft drusen persists without any leakage; the hyperfluorescence of the hard drusen is barely recognizable.

e Color photograph. Geographic atrophy with satellite lesions and pigment clumping, as well as reactive changes in the retinal pigment epithelium.

f Arterial phase. Early filling of the remaining large, deep choroid vessels can be seen as a result of a window defect arising from the loss of the retinal pigment epithelium and choriocapillaris.

g Late phase. Increasing hyperfluorescence in the atrophic area can be seen, concealing the view of the large choroidal vessels. This area of hyperfluorescence has its origins in the hyperfluorescence of the sclera and the window defect as a result of the retinal pigment epithelium atrophy. No leakage is displayed.

h Fundus autofluorescence. The regions with retinal pigment epithelium atrophy show an absence of autofluorescence.

i Fluorescein angiography (in a different patient). Choroidal neovascularization (CNV) after photodynamic therapy. The CNV vessels show hyperfluorescence in the early stage of angiography.

3.2 Age-Related Maculopathy   *Ulrich Kellner*

Epidemiology, Pathophysiology, and Clinical Presentation

- Age-related maculopathy (ARM) is the precursor of age-related macular degeneration (AMD). It is important to identify patients with ARM in order to start prophylactic treatment when appropriate and to inform patients about the symptoms of advanced AMD in order to start treatment as early as possible.
- Drusen are accumulations of protein and lipid-containing amorphous material between the retinal pigment epithelium (RPE) and Bruch membrane.
- On ophthalmoscopy, drusen are visualized as small yellow or white subretinal lesions. A distinction is made between hard and soft varieties of drusen, and mixed forms can also appear. Soft drusen are larger than 65 µm (half the diameter of a vein at the edge of the papilla), and hard drusen are smaller.
- Hard drusen are round, with clearly defined borders; soft drusen are larger, with poorly defined borders, and are partially confluent (medium-sized soft drusen 65–124 µm, large soft drusen > 125 µm).
- The presence of soft, large, and confluent drusen is regarded as a risk factor for progression of the disease. They are sometimes (but not always) associated with impaired vision.
- Hyperpigmentation or hypopigmentation of the retinal pigment epithelium may be present, with variable expression.

Fundus Autofluorescence

- Fundus autofluorescence is a noninvasive method for monitoring progression in age-related maculopathy.
- Not all drusen are visible with fundus autofluorescence.
- Different patterns have recently been classified: normal fundus autofluorescence and increased autofluorescence, with the following patterns: minimal change, focally increased, patchy, linear, lace-like, reticular, and speckled.

Fluorescein Angiography

- On fluorescein angiography, drusen can appear either as hyperfluorescent or hypofluorescent.
- In the early phase of angiography, hard drusen are already visible as hyperfluorescent structures, while in the late phase they tend to show weaker hyperfluorescence.
- Soft drusen accumulate fluorescein more slowly during the course of the angiography. The hyperfluorescence is not as clear, but continues to be present for a longer period in comparison with hard drusen.
- The distinction between confluent soft drusen and a small choroidal neovascularization (CNV) or RPE detachment can be difficult to establish, due to the slow increase in hyperfluorescence.

Diagnosis and Treatment

- The diagnosis can usually be established by binocular ophthalmoscopy. Fundus autofluorescence allows easy monitoring of disease progression. Fluorescein angiography is important in some cases for differentiating between CNV and RPE detachment.
- Providing the patient with information about the symptoms and use of the self-testing Amsler grid are important measures for early detection of the development of exudative AMD and assessing the risk of loss of visual acuity. These are prerequisites for the earliest possible therapy.
- Prophylactic laser coagulation is not a safe treatment option and is associated with a risk of secondary CNV.
- At present, prophylactic treatment with a specific combination of vitamins and nutrient supplements has only been found to be beneficial in relation to disease progression in a subgroup of ARM patients with medium-sized drusen (65–124 µm) and at least one large one (> 125 µm) (ARED study).
- For family members of patients with ARM or AMD who are over the age of 50, a fundus examination is advisable.

References

Age-Related Eye Disease Study Research Group. A randomized, placebo-controlled, clinical trial of high-dose supplementation with vitamins C and E, beta carotene, and zinc for age-related macular degeneration and vision loss: AREDS report no. 8. Arch Ophthalmol 2001;119:1417–36.

Bindewald A, Bird AC, Dandekar SS. Classification of fundus autofluorescence patterns in early age-related macular disease. Invest Ophthalmol Vis Sci 2005,46:3309–14.

Einbock W, Moessner A, Schnurrbusch UE, Holz FG, Wolf S, FAM Study Group. Changes in fundus autofluorescence in patients with age-related maculopathy. Correlation to visual function: a prospective study. Graefes Arch Clin Exp Ophthalmol 2005;243:300–5.

Holz FG, Wolfensberger TJ, Piguet B, et al. Bilateral macular drusen in age-related macular degeneration: prognosis and risk factors. Ophthalmology 1994;101:1522–8.

Hsu J, Maguire MG, Fine SL. Laser prophylaxis for age-related macular degeneration. Can J Ophthalmol 2005;40:320–31.

Sarks JP, Sarks SH, Killingsworth MC. Evolution of soft drusen in age-related macular degeneration. Eye 1994;8:269–83.

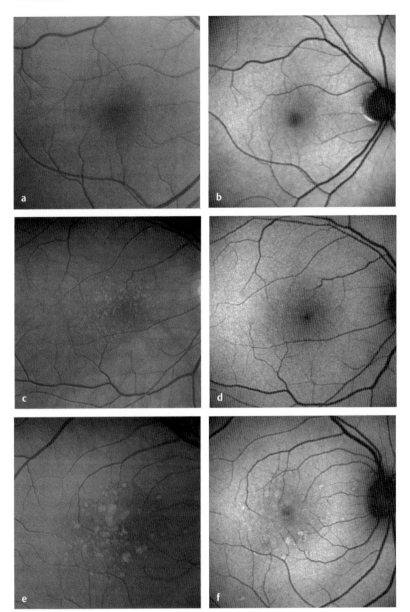

Fig. 3.**2a–f Age-related maculopathy.** Classification of fundus autofluorescence patterns in early age-related macular disease (reproduced with permission from Bindewald et al., Invest Ophthalmol Vis Sci 2005;46:3309–14)

a, b Normal pattern. Homogeneous background fluorescence and a gradual decrease in the inner macula toward the fovea (**b**). Only small hard drusen are visible in the fundus photograph (**a**).

c, d Minimal change pattern. Limited minimal increase or decrease in the intensity of the autofluorescence (**d**) due to multiple small hard drusen (**c**).

e, f Focally increased pattern. Several well-defined spots with markedly increased autofluorescence (**f**) in an eye with multiple soft and hard drusen (**e**).

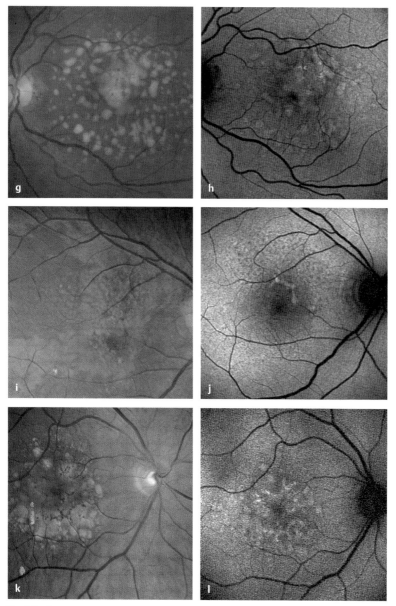

Fig. 3.**2g–l**

g, h Patchy pattern. Multiple large areas (> 200 µm in diameter) of increased autofluorescence (**h**), corresponding to large soft drusen and/or hyperpigmentation (**g**).

i, j Linear pattern. At least one linear area with markedly increased autofluorescence (**j**), corresponding to a hyperpigmented line (**i**).

k, l Lace-like pattern. Multiple branching structures of increased autofluorescence (**l**), corresponding to hyperpigmentation or no visible abnormality on ophthalmoscopy (**k**).

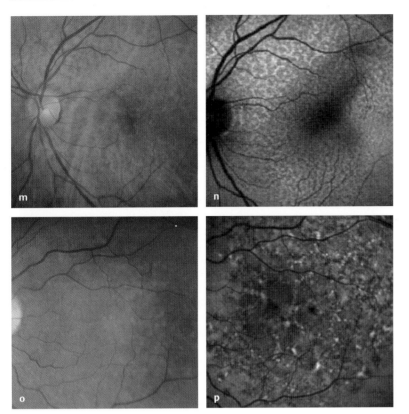

Fig. 3.2m–p

m, n Reticular pattern. Multiple specific areas of decreased auto-fluorescence with brighter lines in between (**n**) may correspond to reticular drusen (**m**).

o, p Speckled pattern. A variety of autofluorescence abnormalities (**p**), whereas the color photograph shows fewer pathological areas (**o**).

3.3 Geographic Atrophy   *Ulrich Kellner*

Epidemiology, Pathophysiology, and Clinical Presentation

- Nonexudative or atrophic age-related macular degeneration ("dry AMD") is one of the two advanced, end-stage types of AMD.
- It mainly involves extended areas with atrophy of the photoreceptors, the retinal pigment epithelium (RPE), and the choriocapillaris, forming a geographic atrophy. Drusen may be present on the edge of the lesion.
- Loss of visual acuity is subtle; individual atrophic areas can, over time, enlarge and become confluent. In bilateral cases, the shape and size of the affected areas are often symmetrical.
- Approximately 20% of severe visual loss in AMD is caused by geographic atrophy.

Fundus Autofluorescence

- The advantages of fundus autofluorescence in comparison with fluorescein angiography are its ability to depict the area surrounding the atrophic zone and its reduced invasiveness for follow-up examinations.
- Fundus autofluorescence makes it possible to depict the atrophic area. Within the atrophic lesion, absence of autofluorescence indicates the loss of RPE and associated lipofuscin. Different, recently classified patterns of abnormal fundus autofluorescence in the junctional zone in geographic atrophy make it possible to draw conclusions regarding the subsequent progression.
- The junctional zone may show either normal autofluorescence, focally increased autofluorescence, a band of increased autofluorescence, patchy increased autofluorescence, or four types of diffusely increased autofluorescence: reticular, branching, fine granular, and fine granular with peripheral punctate spots.

Fluorescein Angiography

- Fluorescein angiography characteristically shows an extended window defect in the area of the atrophy; as a result, a bright hyperfluorescence arises, caused by the abnormally visible choroidal vessel and the fluorescence of the sclera.
- Characteristically, this does not result in visible leakage at the border of the hyperfluorescence. In some cases, the window defect may be confused with choroidal neovascularization or a RPE detachment (see also section 3.1).

Diagnosis and Treatment

- The diagnosis is established clinically, and in some cases angiographically. Fundus autofluorescence examinations allow early detection and assessment of the course of the disease.
- The different patterns of fundus autofluorescence may be associated with different risks of enlargement of the lesion. Preliminary results show that no alterations in the fundus autofluorescence, or only minimal ones, are associated with a lower risk of progression, while increased autofluorescence in the junctional zone indicates areas of progressive RPE loss. Areas of increased autofluorescence are also associated with increased functional loss.
- There are at present no treatment options. Macular translocation is followed by development of geographic atrophy in the new location of the macula. Transplantation of RPE tissue from other areas under the macula is currently being investigated.
- Counseling for visual impairment is advisable, and low-vision aids should be prescribed.

References

Bellmann C, Jorzik J, Spital G, et al. Symmetry of bilateral lesions in geographic atrophy in patients with age-related macular degeneration. Arch Ophthalmol 2002;120:579–84.

Bindewald A, Schmitz-Valckenberg S, Jorzik JJ, et al. Classification of abnormal fundus autofluorescence patterns in the junctional zone of geographic atrophy in patients with age-related macular degeneration. Br J Ophthalmol 2005;89:874–8.

Cahill MT, Mruthyunjaya P, Bowes Rickman C, Toth CA. Recurrence of retinal pigment epithelial changes after macular translocation with 360 degrees peripheral retinectomy for geographic atrophy. Arch Ophthalmol 2005;123:935–8.

Green WR, Enger C. Age-related macular degeneration histopathologic studies. The 1992 Lorenz E. Zimmerman Lecture. Ophthalmology 1993;100:1519–35.

Schmitz-Falkenberg S, Bültmann S, Bindewald A, et al. Fundus autofluorescence and fundus perimetry in the junctional zone of geographic atrophy in patients with age-related macular degeneration. Invest Ophthalmol Vis Sci 2005;45:4470–6.

Sunness JS. The natural history of geographic atrophy, the advanced atrophic form of age-related macular degeneration. Mol Vis 1999;5:25–9.

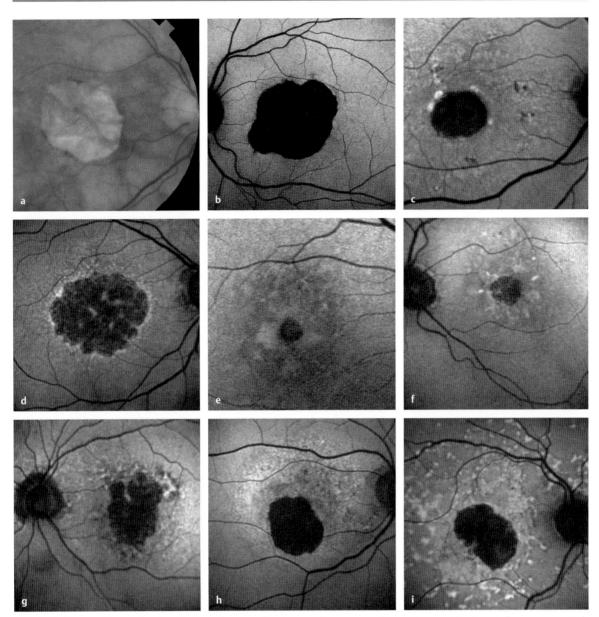

Fig. 3.**3a–i Geographic atrophy.** Classification of abnormal fundus autofluorescence patterns in the junctional zone of geographic atrophy (Figs. 3.**3b–l** reproduced with permission from Bindewald et al., Br J Ophthalmol 2005;89:874–8)

a Fluorescein angiography. Advanced geographic atrophy. The large choroid vessels are visible through the window defect in the retinal pigment epithelium.

b Normal fundus autofluorescence in the junctional zone.

c Multiple patches of markedly focal increased fundus autofluorescence.

d A band of increased fundus autofluorescence surrounding the geographic atrophy.

e Larger areas of patchy increased fundus autofluorescence outside the area of geographic atrophy.

f Diffuse types of increased fundus autofluorescence in the junctional zone of geographic atrophy. Type A: reticular pattern with a preferred radial orientation.

g Type B: increased fundus autofluorescence with short branching linear features.

h Type C: diffusely increased fundus autofluorescence with a fine granular-like appearance surrounding the geographic atrophy.

i Type D: diffusely increased fundus autofluorescence with a fine granular appearance surrounding the geographic atrophy, and peripheral elongated small lesions with increased fundus autofluorescence.

3.4 Classic Choroidal Neovascularization *Joachim Wachtlin*

Epidemiology, Pathophysiology, and Clinical Presentation

- Classic and occult choroidal neovascularization (CNV) have to be distinguished. They can also appear in combined forms; depending on the relative size of the classic part, the condition is described as predominant or minimal classic CNV. Classic CNVs are considerably less frequent than the occult or mixed forms. The common definition in use today is based on the Macular Photocoagulation Study (MPS).
- The diagnosis of a classic CNV requires an angiography. The definition is clinically important, for the choice of therapy. A classic CNV can occur in exudative age-related macular degeneration (AMD), but also secondary to other chorioretinal diseases.
- In addition to actual CNVs, exudative lesions can contain other components, such as fibrosed tissue, hemorrhage, pigmentation, or other features that may obscure the boundaries of the CNV. The term "lesion" can be defined as the entirety of the clinically and angiographically detectable changes, including all of the above-mentioned changes. The distinction between classic and occult and the estimation of size relate to the whole lesion (see also sections 3.7 and 3.13).
- A classic CNV is defined as a clearly visible and well-demarcated hyperfluorescence in the early phase, with increasing leakage in the late phase of the angiography.
- Newly formed fibrovascular networks which grow out of the choriocapillaris through Bruch membrane between the retina and the retinal pigment epithelium (RPE) are the basis for this angiographic picture. In angiography, classic CNVs are therefore better defined than occult CNVs, which principally proliferate under the RPE.
- The initial symptoms of classic CNV are metamorphopsia, deterioration in visual acuity, and central visual field defects.
- Ophthalmoscopic signs of CNV are grayish-white subretinal changes together with retinal edema, hard exudations, and subretinal and intraretinal hemorrhage. If the condition is not treated, progression with enlargement of the lesion and subsequent loss of photoreceptors will usually follow.
- The final stage is a subretinal fibrosis or disciform scar.

Fluorescein Angiography

- An early bright, well-demarcated hyperfluorescence that is caused by vascular proliferations between the RPE and the neuroretina is typical for a classic CNV.
- CNVs appear either as a network with clearly definable vessels or as a homogeneous structure. A small hypofluorescent edge is often visible. Evidence of a clearly defined vascular network is not mandatory for the diagnosis of a classic CNV.
- In the late phase increasing hyperfluorescence with clear leakage is visible, caused by the outflow of dye from the permeable vessels of the CNV.

- Leakage means that the intensity of the hyperfluorescence in the late phase increases and extends beyond the borders of the CNV visible in the early phase.

Diagnosis and Treatment

- A purely clinical distinction between classic and occult CNV is not possible, fluorescein angiography is essential for confirmation and differentiation.
- Angiography is not usually required if exudative changes cannot be clinically detected, if there is extensive hemorrhage, or if a disciform scar can be seen in the advanced form of the disease. In these situations no treatment options exist and the diagnosis can be established without angiography.
- Further categorization of CNVs is based on their position in relation to the center of the fovea (see section 3.7). Treatment recommendations are based on these classifications.
- In subfoveally predominant classic CNVs, photodynamic therapy is the treatment of choice, based on the findings of the Treatment of Age-Related Macular Degeneration with Photodynamic Therapy (TAP) study and Verteporfin in Photodynamic Therapy (VIP) study. In the Macular Photocoagulation Study, the use of argon laser coagulation is reserved for juxtafoveal and extrafoveal classic CNVs (see section 3.12).
- New treatment procedures include intravitreal or subscleral application of agents inhibiting angiogenesis and a combination of photodynamic therapy with either intravitreal application of triamcinolone or angiogenesis-inhibiting agents. The indications for combination treatment and the optimal choice of drug for specific CNV locations or sizes are currently being investigated in detail.
- Optical coherence tomography appears to helpful for treatment control and planning of repeat treatment.

References

Barbazetto I, Burdan A, Bressler NM, et al. Photodynamic therapy of subfoveal choroidal neovascularization with verteporfin: fluorescein angiographic guidelines for evaluation and treatment—TAP and VIP report no. 2. Arch Ophthalmol 2003;121:1253–68.

Grossniklaus HE, Gass JD. Clinicopathologic correlations of surgically excised type 1 and type 2 submacular choroidal neovascular membranes. Am J Ophthalmol 1998;126:59–69.

Krebs I, Binder S, Stolba U, et al. Optical coherence tomography guided retreatment of photodynamic therapy. Br J Ophthalmol 2005;89:1184–7.

Lafaut BA. Clinicopathologic correlation of surgically removed submacular tissue. Bull Soc Belge Ophtalmol 2000;(278):49–53.

Michel S, Wachtlin J, Gamulescu MA, et al. Comparison of early retreatment with the standard regimen in verteporfin therapy of neovascular age-related macular degeneration. Ophthalmology 2005;112:2070–5.

Sarks SH. New vessel formation beneath the retinal pigment epithelium in senile eyes. Br J Ophthalmol 1973;57:951–65.

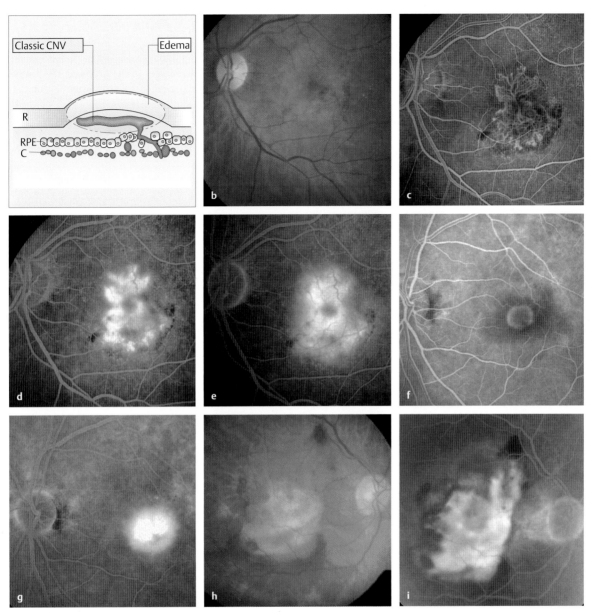

Fig. 3.4a–i Classic choroidal neovascularization

a Schematic representation of the position of a classic choroidal neovascularization between the neuroretina and the retinal pigment epithelium. R, retina; RPE, retinal pigment epithelium; C, choroid.

b Color photograph. The choroidal neovascularization is difficult to identify, and has the appearance of a light gray coloring in the foveal area. Some blood and several drusen are also visible.

c Early arteriovenous phase. The vessel network of the classic choroidal neovascularization appears as an early, well-defined and demarcated hyperfluorescence. It also features several small areas of hypofluorescence resulting from blockage of fluorescence from hemorrhage and hard drusen.

d Late arteriovenous phase. There is a marked increase in hyperfluorescence in the area of the choroidal neovascularization.

e Late phase. Leakage from the choroidal neovascularization. Fluorescein is flowing out of the vessels, and the area of increas-

ing leakage extends beyond the vessel network that was visible in the early phase.

f Early arteriovenous phase. Another example of a classic choroidal neovascularization, consisting of a well-demarcated, homogeneous early hyperfluorescence. However, the vessel loops are not identifiable.

g Late phase. Clear leakage from the choroidal neovascularization is seen.

h Color photograph. The late stage of untreated exudative age-related macular degeneration. An extended disciform scar has formed, with subretinal fibrosis and hemorrhage.

i Late phase. Leakage and staining in the area of the extended fibrosis. This angiogram is not necessary, as the diagnosis could have been established clinically and angiography has no implications for treatment.

3.5 Occult Choroidal Neovascularization   *Faik Gelisken*

Epidemiology, Pathophysiology, and Clinical Presentation

- Occult choroidal neovascularization (CNV) represents a subgroup of neovascular age-related macular degeneration (AMD) and encompasses approximately 80% of all newly diagnosed cases of CNV. Occult CNV is more common in Caucasians and has no gender preference.
- In occult CNV, neovascular vessels from the choroidal capillaries penetrate the Bruch membrane below the retinal pigment epithelium (RPE). Invasion under the retina is also possible when the disease progresses.
- A slow gradual decrease in visual acuity is characteristic of occult CNV (classic CNV is more aggressive).

Fluorescein Angiography

Two types of occult CNV are differentiated angiographically in the Macular Photocoagulation Study (MPS) classification:

- Type 1 (fibrovascular pigment epithelial detachment):
  - Fibrovascular pigment epithelial detachment is the most common form of occult CNV.
  - An irregular elevation of the RPE can be found (stereoscopic fluorescein angiography).
  - In the first few minutes, an inhomogeneous, irregular, increasing hyperfluorescence ("stippled" hyperfluorescence) develops. Subsequently, an increase of hyperfluorescence can be observed (in 5th to 10th minutes).
  - A notch on the edge of an RPE detachment is not a criterion for an occult CNV according to the MPS criteria. However, it does often correlate with the location of an occult CNV.
- Type 2 (late leakage of undetermined source):
  - This type is diagnosed more rarely (partly because of the milder loss of visual acuity, with less exudation) and is more often overlooked as a component of the lesion. There is no RPE detachment.
  - No fluorescein angiographic correlation in the early phase is seen with the late hyperfluorescence.
  - An irregular, inhomogeneous hyperfluorescence can be seen that increases during the late phase of the angiogram.
  - It is often difficult to differentiate between these types of CNV on the basis of an irregular late hyperfluorescence observed around the CNV lesion after photodynamic therapy (PDT).

Additional terminology used in the analysis of CNVs includes the following terms (MPS group and participants in the Verteporfin Round Table):

- Neovascular lesion: the area of the classic and occult choroidal neovascularization.
- Lesion: the whole area of the neovascular lesion and the components of the lesion (e. g., adjacent blood).
- Lesion components: refers to the CNV and the fundus pathologies at the border of the neovascular lesion that obscure the exact borders of the CNV (e. g., pigment, hemorrhage, serous RPE detachment).
- Blocked hyperfluorescence: hypofluorescence caused by blockage on the edge of a neovascular lesion in the absence of a hemorrhage (arising from subretinal fibrin, pigment or subretinal fibrosis). It is classified as a part of the neovascular lesion.
- Predominantly classic or minimally classic CNV: the classic part of the CNV in relation to the neovascular lesion is either more or less than 50%.

Diagnosis and Treatment

- Diagnosis is based on the stereoscopic fluorescein-angiographic classification established by the Macular Photocoagulation Study (MPS).
- It consists of a subretinal fluid or fibrovascular pigment epithelial detachment. Reliable and objective analysis of an occult CNV is only possible using stereoscopic fluorescein angiography.
- Laser coagulation of occult membranes leads to a more unfavorable outcome than the natural course.
- In a subgroup of patients with occult CNVs, photodynamic therapy (PDT) appears to have an advantage over untreated control groups (CNV in less than four disk areas, vision 20/50 or less, recent disease progression). However, in occult CNVs with pigment epithelial detachment, there is a risk of pigment epithelial tears (see section 3.8) with a consequent marked reduction in visual acuity.
- Recently the intravitreal application of Anti-VEGF-agents has shown beneficial effects in selected cases of occult CNV. With the increasing availability of new therapeutic agents (see section 3.14) in the near future the therapy of occult CNV may change rapidly.
- There is currently a lack of established research results for other experimental treatment options (e. g., transpupillary thermo therapy, indocyanine green-guided laser coagulation, feeder vessel occlusion, periocular and intraocular steroid injections, macular surgery).
- A transition between an occult CNV and minimally classic or predominantly classic CNV is possible (50% in 1 year). Despite slowly progressive reductions in visual acuity, therefore, regular examinations with fluorescein angiography are warranted.

References

Barbazetto I, Burdan A, Bressler NM, et al. Photodynamic therapy of subfoveal choroidal neovascularization with verteporfin: fluorescein angiographic guidelines for evaluation and treatment—TAP and VIP report no. 2. Arch Ophthalmol 2003;121:1253–68.

Bressler NM, Frost LA, Bressler SB, Murphy RP, Fine SL. Natural course of poorly defined choroidal neovascularization associated with macular degeneration. Arch Ophthalmol 1988;106:1537–42.

Freund KB, Yannuzzi LA, Sorenson JA. Age-related macular degeneration and choroidal neovascularization. Am J Ophthalmol 1993;115:786–91.

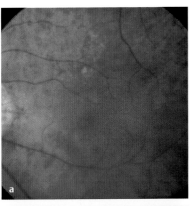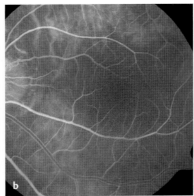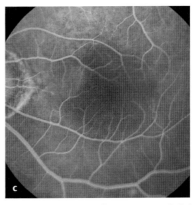

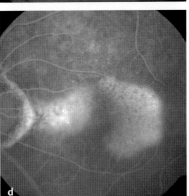

Fig. 3.**5a–d Occult choroidal neovascularization, type 1** (fibrovascular pigment epithelial detachment)

a Color photograph. A flat pigment epithelial detachment is visible in the area of the macula.

b Early arteriovenous phase. An area of hypofluorescence corresponding to the clinically detected fibrovascular pigment epithelial detachment is visible. In contrast to classic choroidal neovascularization, early well-defined hypofluorescence is not seen.

c Arteriovenous phase. Increased hyperfluorescence is visible nasal to the macula. The central and temporal part of the occult choroidal neovascularization still appears hypofluorescent (in this phase, homogeneous hyperfluorescence in the whole lesion would be expected in the case of a purely serous pigment epithelial detachment).

d Late phase. The entire fibrovascular pigment epithelial detachment, up to the fovea, is identifiable with hyperfluorescence in the 5th minute. The irregularity of the border and the inhomogeneous hyperfluorescence are important signs of a fibrovascular pigment epithelial detachment. The kidney-shaped notch also suggests occult choroidal neovascularization.

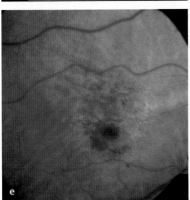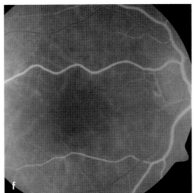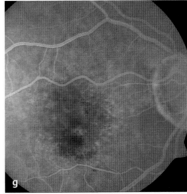

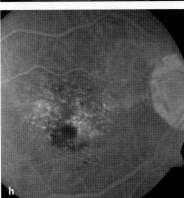

Fig. 3.**5e–h Occult choroidal neovascularization, type 2** (late leakage of undetermined origin)

e Color photograph. A pigment epithelial change in the macular area and subretinal hemorrhage beneath the fovea can be seen.

f Early phase. No hyperfluorescence in the early phase.

g Arteriovenous phase. An ill-defined, inhomogeneous, and irregular area of hyperfluorescence is visible at the macula. A blockage beneath the fovea is caused by subretinal hemorrhage.

h Late phase. Inferotemporal and inferonasal to the fovea, there is an ill-defined area of hyperfluorescence that is inconsistent with the pattern of a pigment epithelial detachment and does not correspond to the early phase of the angiography. No changes can be seen in the early phase that would suggest this hyperfluorescence in the late phase.

Lafaut BA, Bartz-Schmidt KU, Vanden Broecke C, et al. Clinicopathological correlation in exudative age related macular degeneration:
histological differentiation between classic and occult choroidal
neovascularization. Br J Ophthalmol 2000;84:239–43.

Macular Photocoagulation Study Group. Subfoveal neovascular lesions in age-related macular degeneration: guidelines for evaluation and treatment in the Macular Photocoagulation Study. Arch
Ophthalmol 1991;109:1242–57.

Soubrane G, Coscas G, Francais C, Koenig F. Occult subretinal new
vessels in age-related macular degeneration: natural history and
early laser treatment. Ophthalmology 1990;97:649–57.

Verteporfin Roundtable Participants. Guidelines for using verteporfin (Visudyne) in photodynamic therapy for choroidal neovascularization due to age-related macular degeneration and other
causes: update. Retina 2005;25:119–34.

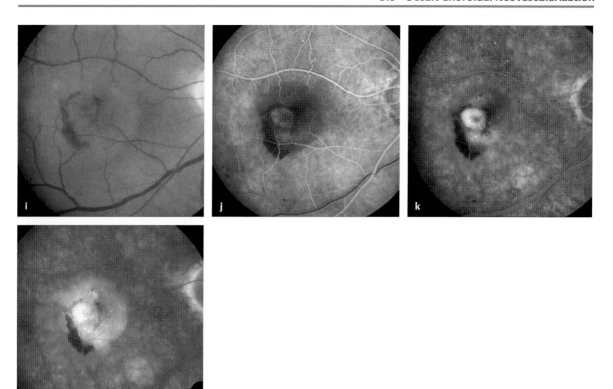

Fig. 3.5i–l   Minimal classic choroidal neovascularization

i   Color photograph. There is subretinal fluid in the macula. A grayish subretinal lesion can be seen temporal to the fovea, surrounded by subretinal hemorrhage.

j   Early phase. A well-defined area of bright hyperfluorescence, consistent with a classic choroidal neovascularization, is visible temporal to the fovea. A blockage is visible, inferior temporal to the classic choroidal neovascularization, which corresponds to the subretinal hemorrhage. In addition, a hypofluorescent ring (which is pronounced inferior of the lesion) can be seen around the classic choroidal neovascularization.

k   Arteriovenous phase. Leakage in the area of the classic choroidal neovascularization. An increasing inhomogeneous disk-shaped area of hyperfluorescence is detectable below and above the classic choroidal neovascularization.

l   Late phase. An intensely leaking lesion can be seen within the disk-shaped inhomogeneous hyperfluorescence. This intensive leakage highlights the classic choroidal neovascularization. The disk-shaped hyperfluorescence is consistent with an occult choroidal neovascularization (type 1; fibrovascular pigment epithelial detachment). There is a subfoveal neovascular lesion with classic and occult components. The classic choroidal neovascularization represents less than 50% of the neovascular lesion (minimally classic choroidal neovascularization).

3.6 Indocyanine Green Angiography in Occult Choroidal Neovascularization *Faik Gelisken*

Indocyanine Green Angiographic Phenomena
Vessel Network of Choroidal Neovascularization

- In choroidal neovascularization (CNV), the vessel network is visible in the early phase. Feeder vessels of the CNV can be detected.
- High-quality images of the vessel network can be obtained with a scanning laser ophthalmoscope and with high-speed indocyanine green (ICG) angiography.

Plaque Hyperfluorescence

- This is a well-defined hyperfluorescence that is often located in the subfoveal area and is larger than one disk diameter.
- Plaque hyperfluorescence is visible in the late phase and represents the less active type or part of occult CNV.
- The best-quality images of plaque hypofluorescence can be obtained using fundus camera-supported angiography systems.

Hot Spots

- A "hot spot" is a well-defined area of focal hyperfluorescence that is smaller than a disk diameter.
- Hot spots are visible in the middle and late phases and represent the active leaking type or part of an occult CNV.
- Hot spots can occur in subgroups of neovascular age-related macular degeneration (AMD), such as retinal angiomatosis proliferation or polypoidal choroidal vasculopathy, and in these cases are usually identifiable in the earlier phases of ICG angiography.

Combined Forms

- More than one ICG angiography characteristics of CNVs can be observed within the same neovascular lesion (e.g., plaque hyperfluorescence with hot spots).
- Laser coagulation of a hot spot can be carried out if it is located extrafoveally or at the edge of a pigment epithelial detachment or plaque hyperfluorescence.

Diagnostic Problems

- Not every area of late hyperfluorescence in ICG angiography is evidence of an occult CNV. Late hyperfluorescence can be observed in some diseases of the choroid—for example, choroidal hemangioma and central serous chorioretinopathy.
- The different ICG angiography systems have various advantages: scanning laser ophthalmoscopes (SLOs) and confocal SLOs are better for detecting choroidal filling in the early phase. Fundus camera-supported systems reveal more sharply defined lesions in the late phase of angiography and are recommended for peripheral fundus lesions.

Advantages of Indocyanine Green Angiography

- Definite diagnosis of a CNV is possible if its vessel network can be identified.
- Differential diagnosis of CNVs in blockages due to subretinal and epiretinal hemorrhage (e.g., macroaneurysms).
- Differentiation of subgroups of AMD, such as polypoidal choroidal vasculopathy and retinal angiomatosis proliferation.
- Differential diagnosis of atypical central serous chorioretinopathy (can mimic an occult CNV, or lead to secondary CNV; see section 8.1). Multiple, well-defined, late, patchy hyperfluorescence at the posterior pole supports the diagnosis of central serous chorioretinopathy.
- Identification of feeder vessels of the CNV, allowing occlusion of the feeder vessels.
- Analysis of the effects of different treatments on the choriocapillaris and choroid (for example, changes in choroidal perfusion following photodynamic therapy, after macular translocation).

Disadvantages of Indocyanine Green Angiography

- The original objective of ICG angiography—to establish a well-defined CNV on the basis of "occult" lesions in fluorescein angiography and thus make occult CNVs accessible for laser coagulation—has not been completely fulfilled.
- The absence of background fluorescence in the early phase makes precise localization of CNVs in relation to the foveal avascular zone difficult.
- The identification of the extent and location of a classic CNV is not sufficiently reliable without additional fluorescein angiography.
- Despite numerous publications on ICG angiography in AMD, the classification and established therapeutic protocols of the CNV are currently based on fluorescein angiography, as defined by the Macular Photocoagulation Study Group.

Implications

- At present, no randomized studies are available on the laser coagulation of hot spots and the occlusion of feeder CNV vessels on the basis of ICG angiography.
- Conventional laser coagulation can be attempted in an extrafoveal or juxtafoveal hot spot in occult CNVs. The results of ICG-guided laser coagulation are comparable, in some studies, with the results reported by the Macular Photocoagulation Study Group in extrafoveal and juxtafoveal well-defined CNVs. However, there has not as yet been a prospective, randomized study of ICG-guided laser treatment of occult CNVs.

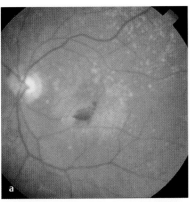

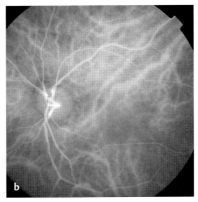

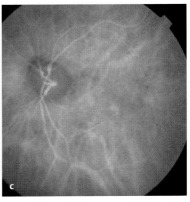

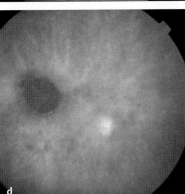

Fig. 3.6a–d Indocyanine green angiography: occult choroidal neovascularization (hot spot)

a Color photograph. Hard and soft drusen in the macula can be seen. Subretinal fluid and a subretinal hemorrhage can be seen inferior to the fovea.

b Indocyanine green angiography, middle phase. No vascular network of choroidal neovascularization is evident. The subretinal hemorrhage beneath the fovea has not produced any blockage.

c Middle phase. Increasing hyperfluorescence beneath the fovea is visible in the 10th minute.

d Late phase. In the 30th minute, a well-defined area of hyperfluorescence beneath the fovea can be seen. The lesion is hyperfluorescent and is smaller than one disk diameter; it is consistent with a hot spot. By definition, the hot spot represents the active part of the occult choroidal neovascularization; it is not detectable in fluorescein angiography, due to blockage by the retinal pigment epithelium or subretinal bleeding.

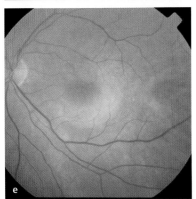

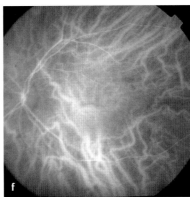

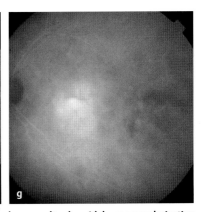

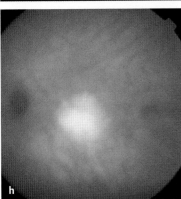

Fig. 3.6e–h Indocyanine green angiography: occult choroidal neovascularization (plaque choroidal neovascularization)

e Color photograph. Subretinal fluid visible in the left eye, at the macula in neovascular age-related macular degeneration.

f Indocyanine green angiography, middle phase. No vessel network of the choroidal neovascularization can be seen.

g Middle phase. Ten minutes after injection of the indocyanine green, there is increased hyperfluorescence resulting from leakage from the occult choroidal neovascularization.

h Late phase. In the 30th minute of indocyanine green angiography, a well-defined subfoveal late hyperfluorescence is visible, which is larger than one disk diameter. This hyperfluorescence represents the nonactive part of an occult choroidal neovascularization—"dormant choroidal neovascularization"—in neovascular age-related macular degeneration.

3

- A hot spot in ICG angiography requires further differential diagnosis from a retinal angiomatosis proliferation, chorioretinal anastomosis, or polypoidal choroidal vasculopathy.
- Conventional laser coagulation of the hot spots has very limited success if it is underlying a pigment epithelial detachment.

References

Geliskin F, Inhoffen W, Schneider U, Stroman GA, Kreissig I. Indocyanine green videoangiography of occult choroidal neovascularization: a comparison of scanning laser ophthalmoscope with high-resolution digital fundus camera. Retina 1998;18:37–43.

Guyer DR, Yannuzzi LA, Ladas I, et al. Indocyanine green-guided laser photocoagulation of focal spots at the edge of plaques of choroidal neovascularization. Arch Ophthalmol 1996;114:693–7.

Guyer DR, Yannuzzi LA, Slakter JS, et al. Classification of choroidal neovascularization by digital indocyanine green videoangiography. Ophthalmology 1996;103:2054–60.

Staurenghi G, Orzalesi N, La Capria A, Aschero M. Laser treatment of feeder vessels in subfoveal choroidal neovascular membranes: a revisitation using dynamic indocyanine green angiography. Ophthalmology 1998;105:2297–305.

Weinberger AW, Knabben H, Solbach U, Wolf S. Indocyanine green guided laser photocoagulation in patients with occult choroidal neovascularization. Br J Ophthalmol 1999;83:168–72.

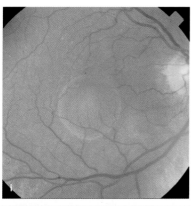
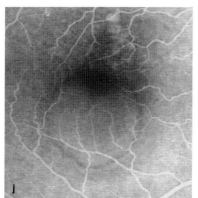
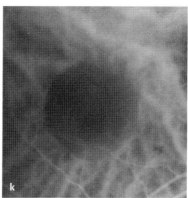
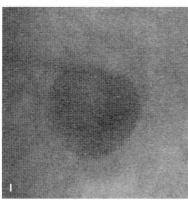

Fig. 3.6i–l Indocyanine green angiography: serous pigment epithelial detachment

i   Color photograph. A sharply-defined elevation can be seen in the macular region, consistent with a serous pigment epithelial detachment.

j   Fluorescein angiography, arteriovenous phase. A disk-shaped area of early hyperfluorescence beneath the macula, involving the fovea, is visible. The homogeneous hyperfluorescence in the early phase is due to staining of the subpigment epithelial fluid by the fluorescein. The hypofluorescence on the upper edge of the pigment epithelial detachment is due to blockage of the xanthophyll pigments in the fovea.

k   Indocyanine green angiography, middle phase. A round, homogeneous area of hypofluorescence matching the extent of the serous pigment epithelial detachment is visible. The hypofluorescence is due to a blockage effect of the subpigment epithelial fluid.

l   Late phase. The serous pigment epithelial detachment is identified in the 30th minute as a persistent hypofluorescent lesion. The absence of any hot spots or plaque hyperfluorescence is an important sign of a nonvascular pigment epithelial detachment.

3

3.7 Localization of Choroidal Neovascularization   *Joachim Wachtlin*

Definitions of Localization

- Choroidal neovascularizations (CNVs) are classified by their position in relation to the avascular center of the fovea. The definition currently in use is based on the Macular Photocoagulation Study (MPS).
  - *Extrafoveal* means that the most central part of the CNV is 200 µm or more from the avascular center of the fovea.
  - *Juxtafoveal* means that the CNV, with its furthest central extension, is between 199 µm and 1 µm from the avascular center of the fovea. The center itself is nevertheless unaffected.
  - *Subfoveal* means that part of the choroidal neovascularization reaches the geometric center of the avascular fovea.

Fluorescein Angiography

- Angiography shows the image of the corresponding CNV (classic/occult or mixed).
- Pure classic CNV should be diagnosed for localization in the early phase of the angiogram (or if appropriate in the early arteriovenous phase). For example, if a vessel network in the early phase shows a juxtafoveal position where increasing leakage continues into the late phase until it reaches the center of the avascular zone (and is therefore subfoveal), then the classic CNV should be categorized as "juxtafoveal." As far as localization is concerned, occult choroidal neovascularizations can only be classified in the late phase of angiography.

- Classifying the location is important for prognosis and possible treatment options in CNV. Research on therapeutic options (laser coagulation and photodynamic therapy) and natural progression depends on this classification.

- The distance from the point of fixation (and therefore the functional center of the fovea) to a choroidal neovascularization can be established clinically, but the classification of the position (subfoveal, juxtafoveal, or extrafoveal) in relation to the avascular center of the fovea is only possible using angiography and may differ.

References

Bird AC, Bressler NM, Bressler SB, et al. An international grading system for age-related maculopathy and age-related macular degeneration. The International ARM Epidemiological Study Group. Surv Ophthalmol 1995;39:367–74.

Macular Photocoagulation Study Group. Argon laser photocoagulation for neovascular maculopathy: five-year results from randomized clinical trials. Arch Ophthalmol 1991;109:1109–14.

Macular Photocoagulation Study Group. Subfoveal neovascular lesions in age-related macular degeneration: guidelines for evaluation and treatment in the Macular Photocoagulation Study. Arch Ophthalmol 1991;109:1242–57.

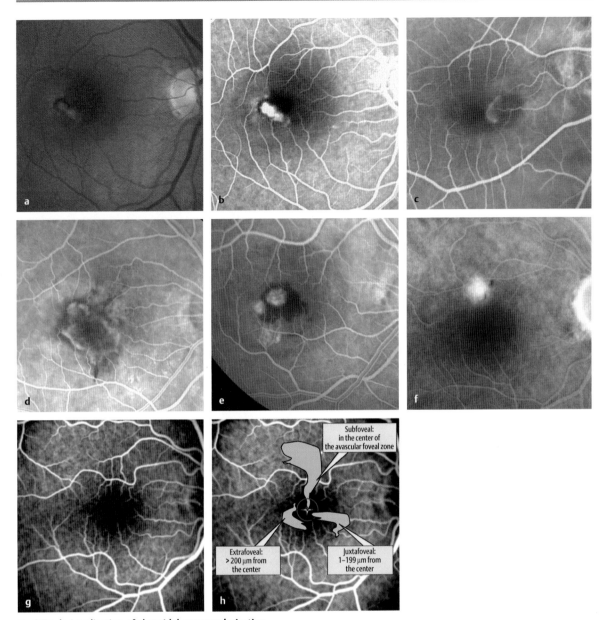

Fig. 3.7a–h Localization of choroidal neovascularization

a Color photograph. The position of the choroidal neovascularization in relation to the avascular center of the fovea is not clearly identifiable.

b Arteriovenous phase. The juxtafoveal position (1–199 μm from the avascular center of the fovea) of the choroidal neovascularization (CNV) is recognizable with angiography. The lesion appears to be a predominantly classic CNV; temporal to the classic component, there is an occult part with increased hyperfluorescence and late leakage.

c Arteriovenous phase (in a different patient). Another example of a classic choroidal neovascularization (CNV) in a juxtafoveal position. The CNV extends into the avascular zone of the fovea, but not into its center.

d Early arteriovenous phase (in a different patient). An example of the extension of a predominantly classic choroidal neovascularization under the avascular center of the fovea, so that the posi-

tion is subfoveal. The occult parts are visible in the temporal direction and above the fovea.

e Arteriovenous phase (in a different patient). The location of the choroidal neovascularization cannot be precisely classified due to blockage resulting from the hemorrhage.

f Late phase (in a different patient). This classic choroidal neovascularization (leakage in the late phase) is located more than 200 μm from the avascular center of the fovea, and is therefore extrafoveal.

g Fluorescence angiography of the avascular areas of the fovea with a normal eye background. The center of the fovea is dark, as there are no retinal capillaries there.

h Schematic representation of the various locations of choroidal neovascularizations or lesions relative to the avascular center of the fovea.

3.8 Pigment Epithelial Tear   *Faik Gelisken*

Epidemiology, Pathophysiology, and Clinical Presentation

- A tear in the retinal pigment epithelium (RPE) may occur in neovascular age-related macular degeneration (AMD).
- Pigment epithelial tears develop due to tangential traction at the edge between attached and detached RPE. An occult choroidal neovascularization (CNV) is often present.
- A pigment epithelial tear may develop as a complication after laser treatment, photodynamic therapy, or transpupillary thermotherapy for neovascular AMD.
- A pigment epithelial tear develops in about 10% of cases with pigment epithelial detachment.
- Frequently, the development of a pigment epithelial tear is associated with to acute visual loss.
- Progressive visual loss in the fellow eye develops in about 80% of cases within 3 years after a pigment epithelial tear in the first eye.

Fluorescein Angiography

- In the acute stage, pigment epithelial tears follow a typical pattern.
- The window defect in the area with absent RPE has a rounded border due to rupture of the pigment epithelium at the edge of the pigment epithelial detachment.
- There is marked hypofluorescence due to increased blockage in the area with the contracted RPE. The edge of this hyperfluorescent area shows a straight border toward the window defect in the acute stage.

Indocyanine Green Angiography

- Hyperfluorescence is seen in the early phase in the area of the RPE tear, which shows isofluorescence in the later phases in indocyanine green angiography.

- Hypofluorescence is present in the area of the contracted RPE.
- Vessels from a choroidal neovascularization or late leakage can be seen in cases of neovascular AMD.

Diagnosis and Treatment

- The diagnosis is made ophthalmoscopically and by fluorescein angiography.
- On ophthalmoscopy, a pigment epithelial detachment with a dark subretinal lesion can be seen. The subretinal structures in the area of the pigment epithelial tear may be less dark. In the acute stage, the border of the tear is clearly visible.
- Fluorescein angiography is the best method of diagnosis in the acute stage. The diagnosis can often not be ascertained in the late stage due to the extensive subretinal fibrosis.
- No definite treatment for pigment epithelial tears is known. In some cases, macular translocation or photodynamic therapy have been reported to have a beneficial effect.

References

Coscas G, Koenig F, Soubrane G. The pretear characteristics of pigment epithelial detachments: a study of 40 eyes. Arch Ophthalmol 1990;108:1687–93.

Gass JD. Pathogenesis of tears of the retinal pigment epithelium. Br J Ophthalmol 1984;68:513–9.

Gelisken F, Schneider U, Inhoffen W, et al. Indocyanine green angiography in retinal pigment epithelial tear. Acta Ophthalmol Scand 1998;76:384–5.

Hoskin A, Bird AC, Sehmi K. Tears of detached retinal pigment epithelium. Br J Ophthalmol 1981;65:417–22.

Schoeppner G, Chuang EL, Bird AC. The risk of fellow eye visual loss with unilateral retinal pigment epithelial tears. Am J Ophthalmol 1989;108:683–5.

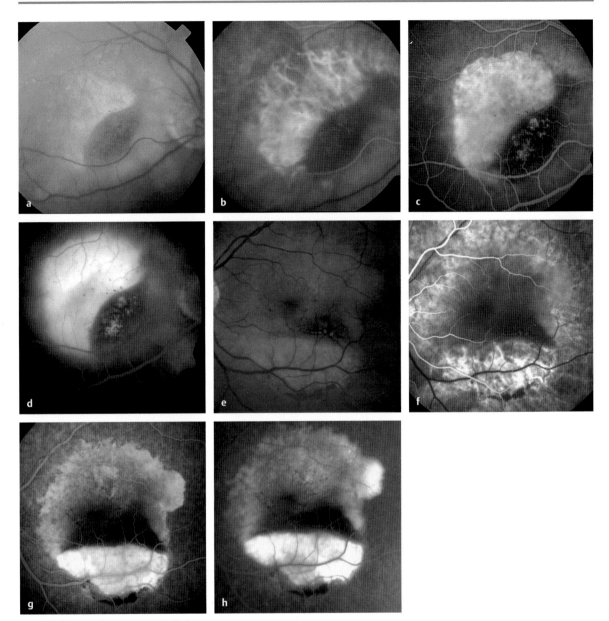

Fig. 3.**8a–h Retinal pigment epithelial tear**

a Color photograph. A hypopigmented area is visible superotemporal to the fovea. Nasal to the fovea, a well-defined oval pigmented lesion can be seen.

b Early arteriovenous phase. Choroidal vessels are visible temporal and above the fovea. This phenomenon is a window defect caused by the lack of the retinal pigment epithelium. Inferior and nasal to the fovea is a blockage caused by the curled retinal pigment epithelium. Around the hypofluorescent and hyperfluorescent lesions, there is homogeneous background fluorescence resulting from intact retinal pigment epithelium.

c Arteriovenous phase. There is an increase in the hyperfluorescence resulting from leakage of the choriocapillaris. In the middle of the blockage, punctate hyperfluorescent spots are seen suggesting a choroidal neovascularization under the contracted retinal pigment epithelium.

d Late phase. There is an increase in the intensity of the hyperfluorescence, consistent with detachment of the neurosensory retina. The fluorescein angiogram findings in this eye are con-

sistent with an acute pigment epithelial tear, caused by an occult choroidal neovascularization on the inferonasal edge of the lesion.

e Color photograph. A pigmented subretinal lesion can be seen under the fovea and inferior to the fovea a sharply demarcated lighter area.

f Early arteriovenous phase. A window defect corresponding to the area of the pigment epithelial tear is visible inferior to the fovea. Above the tear, there is an area of hypofluorescence due to blockage by the contracted retinal pigment epithelium.

g Late arteriovenous phase. Hyperfluorescence in the area of the tear indicates the neurosensory retinal detachment. Above the fovea, the area of hyperfluorescence indicates a fibrovascular pigment epithelial detachment.

h Late phase. Increased hyperfluorescence is visible in the area of the detached neuroretina.

3.9 Retinal Angiomatous Proliferation   *Faik Gelisken*

Epidemiology, Pathophysiology, and Clinical Presentation

- Retinal angiomatous proliferation (RAP) is a newly defined form of exudative maculopathy. As a subgroup of neovascular AMD, it represents 10–15% of newly diagnosed cases, and is frequently bilateral.
- The average age of patients with RAP is 80, with a male–female ratio of 2 : 1.
- The cause of RAP is proliferation of the retinal capillary vessel, with the formation of telangiectases and retinochoroidal anastomoses.
- The process starts secondary to a vascular stimulation in the retina. RAP has to be differentiated from chorioretinal anastomosis in the fibrotic stage of neovascular age-related macular degeneration.
- Treatment of RAP depends on the clinical stage of the disease.

Stages of Retinal Angiomatous Proliferation (Yannuzzi's Classification)

- *Stage I.* Intraretinal neovascularization: extrafoveal retinal proliferation in the capillary vessels, nodular angiomatous growth in the middle and deeper layers of the retina, retinal edema, and intraretinal hemorrhages are seen.
- *Stage II.* Subretinal neovascularization: neovascularization extends into the subretinal area, anastomoses develop between the retinal arterioles and venules, intraretinal edema increases, and retinal, preretinal, and subretinal hemorrhage and serous pigment epithelial detachment occur.
- *Stage III.* Choroidal neovascularization (CNV): clinically or angiographically visible CNV and fibrovascular pigment epithelial detachment; retinochoroidal anastomosis is difficult to detect.

Fluorescein Angiography

- The fluorescein-angiographic characteristics depend on the stage of the RAP:
  - *Stage I.* Paramacular hyperfluorescence caused by retinal leakage and vascular and capillary anomalies in the deeper retina (stereoscopic angiography).
  - *Stage II.* Intraretinal and subretinal hyperfluorescence due to leakage of the retinal and subretinal neovascularizations; hyperfluorescence in the area of the serous pigment epithelial detachment.
  - *Stage III.* Retinochoroidal and retinoretinal anastomoses, hyperfluorescence of the intraretinal and subretinal neovascularizations, and fibrovascular pigment epithelial detachment.

Indocyanine Green Angiography

- Detection of retinochoroidal anastomosis with an associated "hot spot."

- Hypofluorescence of the serous pigment epithelial detachment or filling of the vascular network of the CNV can be seen. Plaque hyperfluorescence can be seen in cases of fibrovascular pigment epithelial detachment.
- There is better detection of retinal vessel anomalies in the presence of preretinal hemorrhage (blockage on fluorescein angiography).

Diagnosis and Treatment

- Signs of retinochoroidal anastomoses that are already clinically evident include an increase in hard exudates and neurosensory detachment in AMD, as well as extrafoveal small intraretinal and preretinal hemorrhage.
- Drusen and pigment epithelial changes similar to AMD can be seen.
- Stereoscopic indocyanine green and fluorescein angiography is helpful in the diagnosis of retinochoroidal anastomosis.
- Precise differentiation from minimal classic CNV is important in stage II (hot spot and serous pigment epithelial detachment).
- The fellow eye of an affected eye should be closely monitored because of the increased risk of developing RAP.
- There is at present no established treatment. Laser coagulation is possible for patients with stage I; photodynamic therapy and macular surgery have been reported for advanced stages of RAP.

References

Borrillo JL, Sivalingam A, Martidis A, Federman JL. Surgical ablation of retinal angiomatous proliferation. Arch Ophthalmol 2003;121:558–61.

Boscia F, Furino C, Sborgia L, et al. Photodynamic therapy for retinal angiomatous proliferations and pigment epithelium detachment. Am J Ophthalmol 2004;138:1077–9.

Hartnett ME, Weiter JJ, Staurenghi G, Elsner AE. Deep retinal vascular anomalous complexes in advanced age-related macular degeneration. Ophthalmology 1996;103:2042–53.

Kuhn D, Meunier I, Soubrane G, Coscas G. Imaging of chorioretinal anastomoses in vascularized retinal pigment epithelium detachments. Arch Ophthalmol 1995;113:1392–8.

Lafaut BA, Aisenbrey S, Vanden Broecke C, Bartz-Schmidt KU. Clinicopathological correlation of deep retinal vascular anomalous complex in age related macular degeneration. Br J Ophthalmol 2000;84:1269–74.

Slakter JS, Yannuzzi LA, Schneider U, et al. Retinal choroidal anastomoses and occult choroidal neovascularization in age-related macular degeneration. Ophthalmology 2000;107:742–54.

Yannuzzi LA, Negrao S, Iida T, et al. Retinal angiomatous proliferation in age-related macular degeneration. Retina 2001;21:416–34.

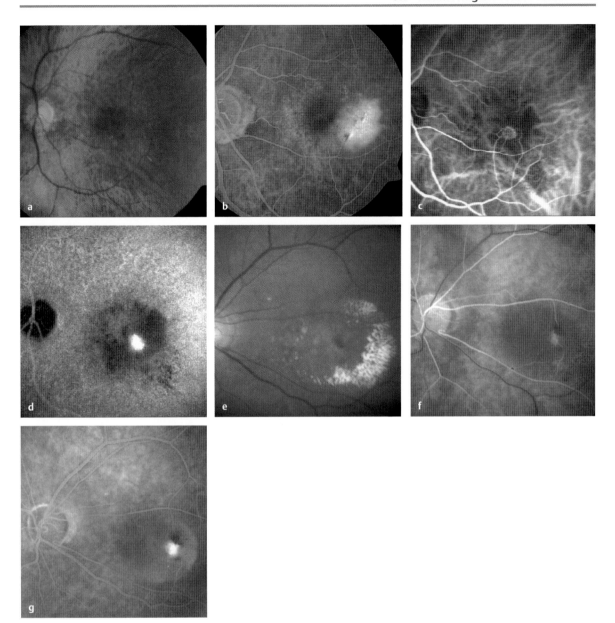

Fig. 3.**9a–g Retinal angiomatous proliferation**

a Color photograph. Drusen and pigment epithelial changes are visible at the macula. A small subretinal hemorrhage and an area of edema are visible temporal to the macula.

b Fluorescein angiography, late phase. An area of hyperfluorescence temporal to the macula is visible, consistent with pigment epithelial detachment. Blockage from the subretinal hemorrhage and a retinal vessel abnormality, presumably an afferent retinal vessel, can be seen inferior and nasal to the pigment epithelial detachment.

c Indocyanine green angiography, middle phase. A well-defined round area of hyperfluorescence is visible, with afferent retinal vessels to this hypofluorescent lesion.

d Late phase. An area of subfoveal hypofluorescence, corresponding to the pigment epithelial detachment, is seen. The well-defined focal hyperfluorescence (hot spot) within the pigment epithelial detachment is due to leakage from the intraretinal and subretinal neovascularization.

e Color photograph. Typical clinical appearance of a RAP lesion with exudates, localized hemorrhage, clinically visible retinal feeder vessels and shallow RPE detachment.

f Early arteriovenous phase. Connection of the classic component of the lesion to two retinal vessels approaching from the superior and inferior aspect of the lesion.

g Late phase. Leakage at the lesion site and the surrounding RPE detachment.

3.10 Polypoidal Choroidal Vasculopathy   *Faik Gelisken*

Epidemiology, Pathophysiology, and Clinical Presentation

- Polypoidal choroidal vasculopathy (PCV) is considered to be a variant of neovascular age-related macular degeneration (AMD), but can also be found in younger patients. The precise definition of the condition—whether it constitutes a subset of AMD, is associated with it, or represents a completely different entity—is currently a matter of debate.
- PCV encompasses approximately 8% of new patients diagnosed with neovascular AMD and is found more commonly in patients of African or Asian origin.
- The pathological changes are mainly located in the inner choroidal vessel network. They are often peripapillary, but can also occur as solitary findings in the macula and periphery.
- Loss of visual acuity originates from subfoveal exudations and hemorrhage. In contrast to pure classic or occult choroidal neovascularization (CNV) secondary to AMD, spontaneous recovery can be observed in a significant proportion of cases.
- Permanent loss of visual acuity occurs due to the subretinal fibrosis and extensive pigment epithelial atrophy at the macula.

Fluorescein Angiography

- Fluorescein angiographic findings depend on the stage of the disease.
- The late phase consists of hyperfluorescence caused by leakage or filling of the polypoidal structures, pigment epithelial detachment, or secondary CNV.
- Occasionally, a subretinal vessel network is visible through the pigment epithelial atrophy.
- In cases of serohemorrhagic pigment epithelial detachment (PED), hyperfluorescence in the superior part of the PED is seen in contrast to the inferior hypofluorescence, caused by to the hemorrhage.

Indocyanine Green Angiography

- The diagnosis is based on indocyanine green (ICG) angiography. A peripapillary pathological vessel network of the choroid and polypoidal hyperfluorescences on the edge of the choroidal vessel network is recognizable in the early phase of ICG angiography.
- In the late phase, ICG washout phenomena are seen in the pathological vessels, and a large area of hyperfluorescence of the neovascular lesion is seen at the macula.

Diagnosis and Treatment

- Clinically, round, small, orange subretinal elevations with subretinal fluid and subretinal hemorrhage are evident. ICG angiography is essential for diagnosis.
- Recurrent multiple serohemorrhagic detachments of the neurosensory retina and the retinal pigment epithelium, usually with a paramacular location, can be observed during the course of the disease.
- In contrast to neovascular AMD, a milder natural course with spontaneous resorption of exudations and hemorrhage and improvement in visual acuity can be observed in a significant proportion of patients.
- However, in the advanced stage of PCV, submacular fibrosis, extensive atrophy of the retinal pigment epithelium and choriocapillaris, as well as pigment migration in the macula, lead to irreversible visual loss.
- There is no approved treatment at present. Patients with extramacular lesions without leakage into the fovea should be observed closely.
- Laser coagulation of the extrafoveal polypoidal lesions can be carried out if the leakage threatens the fovea.
- Photodynamic therapy or macular surgery can be attempted in subfoveal lesions or in progressive macular edema after laser coagulation.

References

Ciardella AP, Donsoff IM, Huang SJ, Costa DL, Yannuzzi LA. Polypoidal choroidal vasculopathy. Surv Ophthalmol 2004;49:25–37.

Costa RA, Navajas EV, Farah ME, Calucci D, Cardillo JA, Scott IU. Polypoidal choroidal vasculopathy: angiographic characterization of the network vascular elements and a new treatment paradigm. Prog Retin Eye Res 2005;24:560–86.

Lafaut BA, Aisenbrey S, Van den Broecke C, Bartz-Schmidt KU, Heimann K. Polypoidal choroidal vasculopathy pattern in age-related macular degeneration: a clinicopathologic correlation. Retina 2000;20:650–4.

Schneider U, Gelisken F, Kreissig I. Indocyanine green angiography and idiopathic polypoidal choroidal vasculopathy. Br J Ophthalmol 1998;82:98–9.

Yannuzzi LA, Sorenson J, Spaide RF, Lipson B. Idiopathic polypoidal choroidal vasculopathy (IPCV). Retina 1990;10:1–8.

Yannuzzi LA, Wong DW, Sforzolini BS, et al. Polypoidal choroidal vasculopathy and neovascularized age-related macular degeneration. Arch Ophthalmol 1999;117:1503–10.

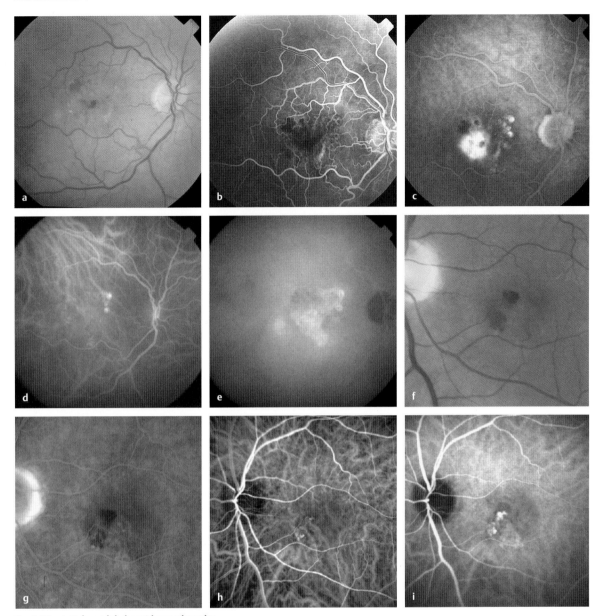

Fig. 3.10a–i Polypoidal choroid vasculopathy

a Color photograph. Subretinal hemorrhage, macular edema, and lipid deposits can be seen temporal to the macula.

b Fluorescein angiography, arteriovenous phase. Multiple, round areas of hyperfluorescence are seen nasal to the macula. The center of these polypoidal lesions is still hypofluorescent. An area of hypofluorescence secondary to blockage by subretinal hemorrhage can be seen in the macula. An area of hyperfluorescence can be seen nasally and beneath the fovea, suggesting leakage from the subretinal vasculopathy.

c Late phase. Polypoidal lesions are visible nasal to the macula, with increasing hyperfluorescence. Leakage at the macula is also present.

d Indocyanine green angiography, middle phase. Hyperfluorescent polypoidal lesions are seen superior and nasal to the fovea.

e Late phase. After wash-out of the indocyanine green, the entire lesion appears as a large area of hyperfluorescence at the macula.

f Color photograph. Hemorrhagic maculopathy in the left eye.

g Fluorescein angiography, late phase. Blockages caused by subretinal hemorrhages can be seen nasal to the fovea, and a poorly defined area of hyperfluorescence is visible inferior and nasal to the fovea.

h Indocyanine green angiography, middle phase. Multiple, round areas of hyperfluorescence are recognizable nasal and inferior to the fovea.

i Late phase. The polypoidal choroid vasculopathy can be seen, with two hot spots and a late area of hyperfluorescence inferonasal to the fovea.

3.11 Choroidal Neovascularization: Other Etiologies   *Joachim Wachtlin*

Introduction

- Age-related macular degeneration is the most common cause of the development of choroidal neovascularization (CNV). In order of frequency, other causes include:
  – Myopia
  – Post-inflammatory conditions, e. g. after chorioretinitis
  – Idiopathic
  – Angioid streaks, trauma, macular dystrophy, etc.
- Most commonly, disintegration of the functional complexes of the choroid, the retinal pigment epithelium (RPE), Bruch membrane, and the choriocapillaris takes place. In a second step, a CNV can develop—usually a classic CNV.

Myopia

- Pathological myopia (axial length > 25 mm or refraction > –6.0 D) can results in the development of myopic maculopathy.
- Myopic maculopathy encompasses macular chorioretinal atrophy and lacquer cracks (tears in Bruch membrane).
- Hemorrhage can occur in the lacquer cracks and can sometimes be associated with CNV.
- If untreated, a slightly prominent pigmented scar in the fovea—the Fuchs spot—can result.

Postinflammatory Choroidal Neovascularization

- Various inflammatory diseases can lead to the development of a CNV.
- Histoplasmosis is a systemic infection with the fungus *Histoplasma capsulatum* that is endemic mainly in the Mississippi and Missouri region. Ocular histoplasmosis syndrome (OHS) develops in a proportion of these patients.
- Typical clinical findings for ocular histoplasmosis syndrome are: peripapillary choroidal atrophy, histospots (small punched-out scars), in some cases CNV, but no intraocular inflammation.
- As *Histoplasma capsulatum* is not endemic in Europe, a clinically identical disease entity termed presumed ocular histoplasmosis syndrome (POHS) has been defined.
- Other rare chorioretinal inflammations that can lead to CNV are:
  – Punctate inner choroidopathy (PIC), with small, indistinct yellow spots (mainly in young myopic women).
  – Multifocal choroiditis with panuveitis (MFCP), similar to presumed ocular histoplasmosis syndrome, but with vitreitis.

Additional Causes of Choroidal Neovascularization

- Idiopathic CNV is a diagnosis of exclusion, if there are no signs of age-related macular degeneration or age-related maculopathy (drusen), no other cause of CNV is evident, and the patient is under the age of 50. The disease is often bilateral. The pathogenesis usually remains undetermined.

- In angioid streaks, tears form in Bruch membrane, combined with subretinal fibrosis and CNV with a bad prognosis. This disease entity is often associated with pseudoxanthoma elasticum (see section 8.6).
- In traumatic choroidal ruptures, the CNV develops on the edge of the rupture (see section 8.6).
- CNV rarely occurs in patients with hereditary macular dystrophy.

Diagnosis and Treatment

- The diagnosis of the underlying disease entity is carried out clinically, while the CNV is defined by fluorescein angiography.
- When the lesion has a juxtafoveal and extrafoveal location in patients with ocular histoplasmosis syndrome and myopia, argon laser coagulation is a possible treatment option, as used in the MPS study. This type of CNV can also be treated successfully with photodynamic therapy (PDT).
- In subfoveal locations in OHS and myopia, treatment with PDT promises the best results at present (VIP study).
- There have as yet not been any controlled studies on presumed ocular histoplasmosis syndrome (POHS); patients are treated in a similar way to those with OHS.
- Enlargement of laser scars after the treatment of CNVs that were not caused by age-related macular degeneration should be taken into consideration when discussing therapeutic options. PDT can therefore also be considered in juxtafoveal locations in these patients.
- Natural progression and subretinal surgery are associated with a better prognosis mainly in idiopathic CNVs, rather than in age-related macular degeneration, as the extent of the damage to the RPE appears to be comparatively less.

References

Avila MP, Weiter JJ, Jalkh AE, Trempe CL, Pruett RC, Schepens CL. Natural history of choroidal neovascularization in degenerative myopia. Ophthalmology 1984;91:1573–81.

Blinder KJ, Blumenkranz MS, Bressler NM, et al. Verteporfin therapy of subfoveal choroidal neovascularization in pathologic myopia: 2-year results of a randomized clinical trial—VIP report no. 3. Ophthalmology 2003;110:667–73.

Macular Photocoagulation Study Group. Argon laser photocoagulation for neovascular maculopathy: five-year results from randomized clinical trials. Macular Photocoagulation Study Group. Arch Ophthalmol 1991;109:1109–14.

Parnell JR, Jampol LM, Yannuzzi LA, Gass JD, Tittl MK. Differentiation between presumed ocular histoplasmosis syndrome and multifocal choroiditis with panuveitis based on morphology of photographed fundus lesions and fluorescein angiography. Arch Ophthalmol 2001;119:208–12.

Saperstein DA, Rosenfeld PJ, et al. Photodynamic therapy of subfoveal choroidal neovascularization with verteporfin in the ocular histoplasmosis syndrome: one-year results of an uncontrolled, prospective case series. Ophthalmology 2002;109:1499–505.

Wachtlin J, Heimann H, Behme T, Foerster MH. Long-term results after photodynamic therapy with verteporfin for choroidal neovascularizations secondary to inflammatory chorioretinal diseases. Graefes Arch Clin Exp Ophthalmol 2003;241:899–906.

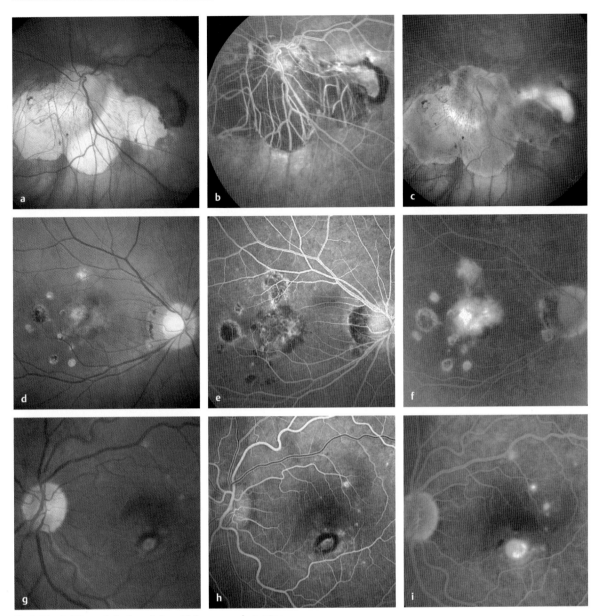

Fig. 3.11a–i Other etiologies of choroidal neovascularization

a   Color photograph. Myopia with retinochoroidal atrophy and posterior staphyloma in high myopia. The sclera is visible through choroidal defects. A gray edematous area with hemorrhage is located on the temporal edge of the staphyloma and the atrophy.

b   Arteriovenous phase. An area of hypofluorescence appears in the area of the choroidal atrophy, due to absent perfusion of the choriocapillaris. Single choroidal vessels are visible next to retinal vessels. An area of early hyperfluorescence is visible on the edge, resulting from the choroidal neovascularization, surrounded by a blockage from the hemorrhage.

c   Late phase. An area of hyperfluorescence is now visible near the atrophy, resulting from background fluorescence from the sclera. There is now clear leakage in the area of the choroidal neovascularization.

d   Color photograph. Typical small punched-out scars (histospots) are recognizable in a patient with presumed ocular histoplasmosis syndrome. Adjacent to the small scars, peripheral atrophy and an exudative maculopathy with hemorrhage can also be seen.

e   Arteriovenous phase. An area of early hyperfluorescence corresponding to a choroidal neovascularization is visible centrally. Blockage phenomena are recognizable in the area of the scars, hemorrhage, and pigmentations.

f   Late phase. Leakage from the choroidal neovascularization. The nonpigmented scars show hyperfluorescence as window defects; the pigmented scars only show a hyperfluorescent edge.

g   Color photograph. In punctate inner choroidopathy, small yellow–white spots with ill-defined borders can be seen in the choroid at the posterior pole.

h   Early phase. Early hyperfluorescence of the spots can be seen, in contrast to the scars associated with presumed ocular histoplasmosis syndrome. In addition, a juxtafoveal area of hyperfluorescence can be observed, surrounded by a hypofluorescent edge.

i   Late phase. Continued increase in hyperfluorescence in the individual spots. In addition, there is a mildly active juxtafoveal choroidal neovascularization with only minor leakage and staining.

3.12 Angiography after Laser Treatment for Choroidal Neovascularization   *Faik Gelisken*

Laser Photocoagulation: Principle and Research

- The principle of laser photocoagulation consists of thermal destruction of a choroidal neovascularization (CNV). As a consequence, the overlying photoreceptors and the retinal pigment epithelium (RPE) are destroyed in the treated areas.
- The Macular Photocoagulation Study Group (MPS) demonstrated the beneficial effects of laser coagulation of juxtafoveal and extrafoveal classic CNVs in reducing the risk of severe visual loss.
- Occult or ill-defined CNVs should not be treated with argon laser, as incomplete treatment leads to a higher risk of recurrence and progression of the CNV.
- Argon laser coagulation of subfoveal CNVs leads to an acute decrease in visual acuity immediately after laser treatment, and a noticeable statistical advantage over the natural course is only observed after 2 years of long-term follow-up. According to the MPS group, patients with small CNV lesions who initially have poor vision have a better functional outcome than those with CNV lesions with better vision after laser treatment. Because of the acute visual loss after, laser coagulation of subfoveal classic CNV has not been widely accepted in clinical practice.
- The recurrence rate after laser photocoagulation is up to 50% of cases within 2 years; recurrences are often subfoveal.

Fluorescein Angiography

- Following laser treatment, eyes with CNVs should be monitored with fluorescein angiography after 2 and 6 weeks, and thereafter at 3-monthly intervals for the first year.

- In the early phase of fluorescein angiography, a round area of hypofluorescence is observed, indicating a filling defect resulting from closure of the choriocapillaris by laser photocoagulation. A circular area of hyperfluorescence can be seen on the edge of the hypofluorescence. This phenomenon is due to a window defect, caused by depigmentation of the RPE (due to collateral damage by laser coagulation) and the consequent visibility of fluorescein in the choriocapillaris.
- In cases with a dry laser scar, the borders of the laser-scar indicated by hyperfluorescence in the early and late phases of the fluorescein angiogram remain the same and display no leakage.
- By contrast, recurrent or persistent CNVs present with progressive hyperfluorescence due to leakage from the CNV.

References

Barbazetto I, Burdan A, Bressler NM, et al. Photodynamic therapy of subfoveal choroidal neovascularization with verteporfin: fluorescein angiographic guidelines for evaluation and treatment—TAP and VIP report no. 2. Arch Ophthalmol 2003;121:1253–68.

Macular Photocoagulation Study Group. Subfoveal neovascular lesions in age-related macular degeneration: guidelines for evaluation and treatment in the Macular Photocoagulation Study. Arch Ophthalmol 1991;109:1242–57.

Macular Photocoagulation Study Group. Laser photocoagulation of subfoveal neovascular lesions of age-related macular degeneration: updated findings from two clinical trials. Arch Ophthalmol 1993;111:1200–9.

Macular Photocoagulation Study Group. Laser photocoagulation for juxtafoveal choroidal neovascularization: five-year results from randomized clinical trials. Arch Ophthalmol 1994;112:500–9.

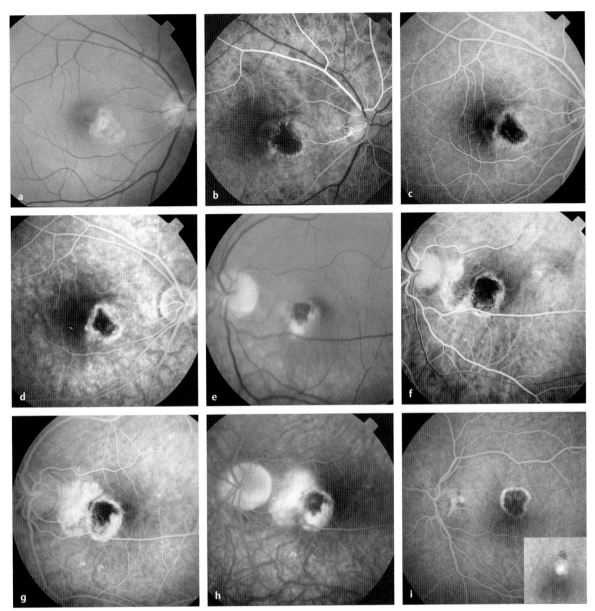

Fig. 3.12a–i Angiography after laser treatment for choroidal neovascularization

a Color photograph. Laser photocoagulation for an extrafoveal choroidal neovascularization. Nasal to the fovea, a hypopigmented lesion and subretinal fibrosis are visible. A small subretinal hemorrhage can be seen in the fovea.

b Early phase. A round area of hypofluorescence, indicating a filling defect from the laser photocoagulation. The hyperfluorescence on the border of the hypofluorescence corresponds to the visible fluorescein in the choriocapillaris, transmitted through the pigment epithelial defects on the edge of the laser scar.

c Arteriovenous phase. Extrafoveal hypofluorescence, indicating a dry laser scar.

d Late phase. The laser scar is still dry. The hyperfluorescence follows the borders established in the early phase of the fluorescein angiography, and matches the pigment epithelial defect.

e Color photograph. Previous laser photocoagulation of an extrafoveal choroidal neovascularization. An atrophic pigmented laser scar can be seen nasal to the fovea. Accumulation of subretinal fluid and a gray subretinal lesion are present nasally and above the laser scar.

f Early arteriovenous phase. A round, hypofluorescent laser scar can be seen nasal to the fovea, surrounded by a hyperfluorescent border. The vascular network of a recurrent choroidal neovascularization with a feeder vessel is visible at the nasal border of the laser scar.

g Middle arteriovenous phase. The details of the choroidal neovascularization network are not detectable due to increased leakage.

h Late phase. Increased hyperfluorescence is visible, covering the edges of the recurrent choroidal neovascularization.

i Classic extrafoveal choroidal neovascularization after laser coagulation. Inset: extrafoveal choroidal neovascularization, with leakage before coagulation. Main image: central hypofluorescence from the filling defect and the hyperfluorescent edge of the laser scar in the late phase. There is no leakage from the laser scar, which would indicate recurrent choroidal neovascularization.

3.13 Angiography after Photodynamic Therapy for Choroidal Neovascularization *Joachim Wachtlin*

Photodynamic Therapy: Principle and Research

- Photodynamic therapy is currently the treatment of choice for subfoveal classic or predominantly classic choroidal neovascularizations (CNV) in age-related macular degeneration.
- A photosensitizing agent is administered intravenously, which accumulates in the CNV and is selectively activated with a special laser. Highly reactive oxygen compounds develop that lead to thrombosis of the CNV. Retinal vessels in the treatment area are not subject to thrombosis.
- Large controlled studies—the Treatment of Age-Related Macular Degeneration with Photodynamic Therapy (TAP) study and Verteporfin in Photodynamic Therapy (VIP) study—have shown that in age-related macular degeneration with subfoveal, predominantly classic choroidal neovascularization, a loss of visual acuity of 3 or more lines can be prevented with photodynamic therapy in a significant proportion of patients, in comparison with placebo groups.
- More recent studies have also shown that the treatment is effective in small occult CNVs and CNVs arising due to other diseases.
- In principle, PDT is also effective for juxtafoveal and extrafoveal CNVs.
- Further investigations have shown that small lesions have a better overall prognosis in relation to visual acuity than larger ones.
- The indications for PDT, as well as reimbursement for it by health insurance companies, are constantly changing. Physicians therefore need to obtain current information from the appropriate administrative bodies.
- As the treatment generally needs to be repeated regularly, it is clinically important for physicians to be familiar with the characteristic angiographic results after PDT.
- Typical changes after PDT include secondary pigmentations and what is known as staining.
- The typical fundamental changes in CNVs observed after photodynamic therapy should also be assessed after combination therapy (PDT and triamcinolone or PDT and Anti-VEGF treatment).

Fluorescein Angiography
Hypofluorescence

- Immediately after PDT, the choriocapillaris shows temporarily reduced perfusion. As a result, up to approximately 4–6 weeks after treatment, a hypofluorescent area is visible in the treatment region.
- Usually, no further hypofluorescence can be detected 6 weeks after treatment.

Leakage

- New leakage can occur during the clinical course after PDT as a result of reperfusion of the CNV or recurrent CNV. The size and composition (classic or occult) of the CNV can change.
- Leakage and recurrent or persistent metamorphopsia generally indicate that further PDT treatment is required. In larger studies, an average of three or four treatment cycles are carried out per patient in the first year.

Pigmentation

- Stronger pigmentation around the CNV is visible particularly after repeated PDT and in younger patients; in these cases, the retinal pigment epithelial cells envelop the CNV.
- Pigmentation leads, due to blockage, to hypofluorescence on the border of the CNV.

Staining

- Staining represents a slight increase in hyperfluorescence in the scarred or fibrotic areas and is identifiable as an area of hyperfluorescence without leakage or retinal edema.
- After repeated PDT, argon laser coagulation, or in the end stages of AMD, staining is often visible with subretinal fibrosis and scaring, and is difficult to differentiate from leakage.
- A small increase in hyperfluorescence up to approximately 5 min after injection is typical. A decrease in hyperfluorescence is generally detectable up to the 10th minute.
- In contrast, the intensity of the hyperfluorescence, indicating leakage, remains constant or increases between the 5th and 10th minutes of the angiography.
- With staining, the hyperfluorescent area in the late phase does not go beyond the boundaries of the lesion detected in the early phase.
- In addition to the fluorescein-angiographic findings, clinical assessment of exudative changes should also be carried out. Additional information can be obtained from stereo angiography. Alternatively, the angiographic findings have to be correlated with the binocular ophthalmoscopic findings. Optical coherence tomography is also helpful in these situations and is being used more frequently for observation after PDT.
- With staining, there is no indication for further PDT treatment. However, leakage suggests a persisting or recurrent CNV, and further treatment should therefore be discussed.

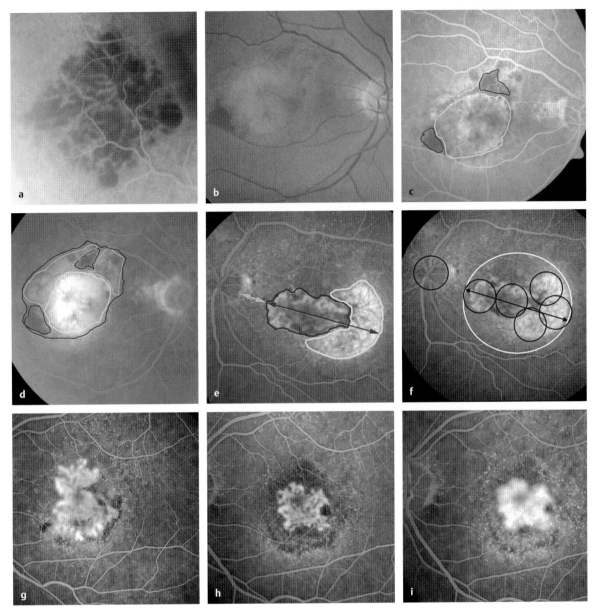

Fig. 3.13a–i Angiography after photodynamic therapy for choroidal neovascularization

a Early arteriovenous phase. The result 3 days after experimental photodynamic therapy. A definite area of hypoperfusion in the choriocapillaris is visible; the large choroidal vessels are perfused. The retinal vessels show no change in perfusion.

b Color photograph. A grayish-white lesion can be seen in the macula, with hemorrhage at the border. No clear-cut diagnosis or differentiation of the choroidal neovascularization (CNV) can be made.

c Arteriovenous phase. The classic part of the lesion (the yellow-bordered area) can be seen as an early definable hyperfluorescence with two small hemorrhages (the red-bordered area), which lead to a blockage and hypofluorescence.

d Late phase. An occult part of the CNV (the green-bordered area), with hyperfluorescence and leakage with clear origins in the late phase, is also definable. The blue-bordered area shows that the whole lesion consists of CNV (classic and occult) and other components of a choroidal neovascular lesion.

e Angiography with important treatment parameters for the indications for and implementation of photodynamic therapy. Red:

the classic part of the CNV; yellow: the occult part of the CNV; blue: largest linear diameter of the CNV; light blue: distance to the optic nerve head.

f Angiography, with schematic representation of the parameters of a CNV. Black circle: one optic disc diameter; black arrow: largest linear diameter of the CNV. The CNV has a diameter of approximately 5200 μm and a minimum surface area of 5 optic disc diameters.

g Arteriovenous phase (in a different patient). A classic subfoveal CNV before photodynamic therapy. A clearly demarcated area of early hyperfluorescence with developing leakage is recognizable.

h Arteriovenous phase. Six weeks after photodynamic therapy (PDT), the CNV is clearly smaller. Near the treatment spots, there is an area of mild hypofluorescence resulting from the decreased perfusion after PDT.

i Late phase. There is still leakage, indicating that further treatment is required.

References

Barbazetto I, Burdan A, Bressler NM, et al. Photodynamic therapy of subfoveal choroidal neovascularization with verteporfin: fluorescein angiographic guidelines for evaluation and treatment—TAP and VIP report no. 2. Arch Ophthalmol 2003;121:1253–68.

Blinder KJ, Bradley S, Bressler NM, et al. Effect of lesion size, visual acuity, and lesion composition on visual acuity change with and without verteporfin therapy for choroidal neovascularization secondary to age-related macular degeneration: TAP and VIP report no. 1. Am J Ophthalmol 2003;136:407–18.

Bressler NM. Verteporfin therapy of subfoveal choroidal neovascularization in age-related macular degeneration: two-year results of a randomized clinical trial including lesions with occult with no classic choroidal neovascularization—verteporfin in photodynamic therapy report 2. Am J Ophthalmol 2002;133:168–9.

Kaiser RS, Berger JW, Williams GA, et al. Variability in fluorescein angiography interpretation for photodynamic therapy in age-related macular degeneration. Retina 2002;22:683–90.

Michels S, Schmidt-Erfurth U. Sequence of early vascular events after photodynamic therapy. Invest Ophthalmol Vis Sci 2003;44:2147–54.

TAP Study Group. Photodynamic therapy of subfoveal choroidal neovascularization in age-related macular degeneration with verteporfin: one-year results of 2 randomized clinical trials—TAP report. Treatment of age-related macular degeneration with photodynamic therapy (TAP) Study Group. Arch Ophthalmol 1999;117:1329–45.

Verteporfin Roundtable Participants. Guidelines for using verteporfin (Visudyne) in photodynamic therapy for choroidal neovascularization due to age-related macular degeneration and other causes: update. Retina 2005;25:119–34.

Wachtlin J, Stroux A, Wehner A, Heimann H, Foerster MH. Photodynamic therapy with verteporfin for choroidal neovascularizations in clinical routine outside the TAP study: one- and two-year results including juxtafoveal and extrafoveal CNV. Graefes Arch Clin Exp Ophthalmol 2005;243:438–45.

3

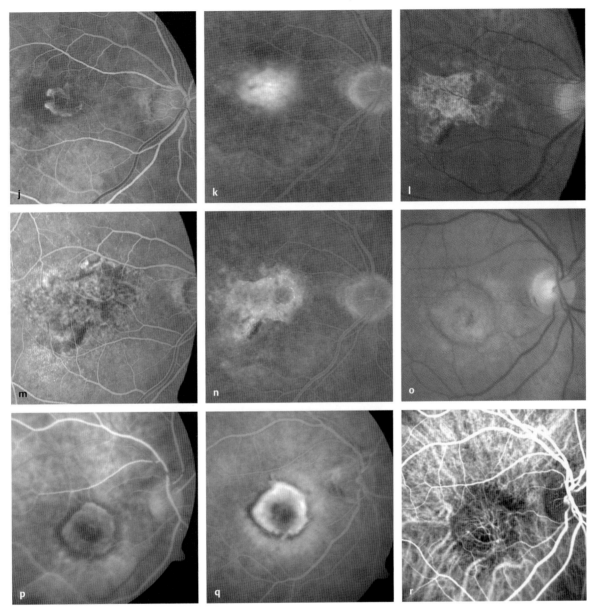

Fig. 3.13j–r Angiography after photodynamic therapy for choroidal neovascularization

j Arteriovenous phase (in a different patient). A predominantly classic choroidal neovascularization (CNV) before photodynamic therapy.

k Late phase. Active leakage from the predominantly classic CNV.

l Color photograph of the eyes in **j** and **k**. Two years after the initial photodynamic therapy, a total of three treatment sequences were carried out. Yellow, partly light-pigmented subretinal fibrosis is visible.

m Arteriovenous phase. Some areas show limited mild hyperfluorescence; there is hypofluorescence in the area in which the fibrosis is more strongly pigmented.

n Late phase. Only minimal fluorescence appears in the retinal and choroid vessels in the late phase. The clinically visible fibrosis presents as a clear, well-defined hyperfluorescent area. The fluorescein only accumulates slowly in the fibrotic tissue. In contrast to an active lesion with leakage, the hyperfluorescent area has exactly the same dimensions as the ophthalmoscopically visible fibrosis and does not show any leakage beyond the borders of the fibrosis.

o Color photograph. Subretinal fibrosis after photodynamic therapy, with a pigmented border and with no retinal edema.

p Early arteriovenous phase. An area of early hyperfluorescence with a hypofluorescent border is seen. The borders and size of the lesion correspond precisely to the lesion visualized in the color photograph.

q Late phase. The hyperfluorescence in the scar area has marginally increased, but has not extended beyond the clearly marked borders of the lesion visible in the early phase. There is no leakage, and only staining is present in the scar.

r Indocyanine green angiography. Within the CNV, a few perfused vessels with fibrotic changes show very minimal perfusion, without leakage.

3.14 Angiography after Intravitreal Drug Administration for Choroidal Neovascularization   *Ulrich Kellner and Joachim Wachtlin*

Antiangiogenesis: Principle and Research

- Laser treatment and photodynamic therapy (PDT) can be only be carried out in a limited number of patients with neovascular age-related macular degeneration. The search for new treatment options has resulted in the development of several drugs that affect the events leading to new vessel formation (angiogenesis). Some drugs inhibit the action of vascular endothelial growth factor (VEGF) directly, whereas other drugs inhibit protein kinase C or other factors involved in the neovascular process.
- Pegaptanib sodium (Macugen), a ribonucleic acid aptamer that binds to the extracellular VEGF-165 amino acid isoform, is currently available. At present, intraocular injections every 6 weeks are recommended.
- Drugs currently being investigated include the following:
  - Ranibizumab (Lucentis) is a small antibody fragment that binds all isoforms of VEGF. Intravitreal injections every 4 weeks are being used in clinical trials. Ranibizumab has shown improvement of visual acuity in small studies. It is expected to be available in 2006.
  - Bevacizumab (Avastin), a larger anti-VEGF monoclonal antibody of which ranibizumab is a fragment, is presently available for cancer treatment. In a small study, systemic application of bevacizumab has been shown to be effective as well. Side effects of the systemic treatment and the availability of the drug have induced a recent increase of intravitreal application of bevacizumab. Long-term follow-up and results from randomized studies do not exist.
  - Anecortave acetate (Reetane) is an angiostatic cortisone that lacks the glucocorticoid-mediated side effects of corticosteroids. The agent's effect is due to inhibition of plasminogen activators and matrix metalloproteinases, which are mandatory for endothelial-cell proliferation. Posterior juxtascleral depot injection with a special needle every 6 months is being used in clinical trials.
  - Triamcinolone acetonide has a limited antiangiogenetic effect, but has a marked anti-inflammatory effect due to mediators such as prostaglandins or leukotrienes. Triamcinolone has been injected intravitreally for a multitude of macular disorders. Its efficacy in the treatment of choroidal neovascularization has only been demonstrated in combination with PDT. Side effects include increased ocular pressure and cataract formation. Recently, juxtascleral injection in combination with PDT has been reported. Intravitreal injection of triamcinolone acetate is not an approved application of the drug in many countries, and physicians are therefore recommended to clarify the legal status with the appropriate local authorities.

- With the exception of the various application regimens, experience with these drugs is limited to a few research studies, and the advantages of or specific indications for any of the drugs in different forms of AMD have yet to established.
- The drugs also appear to be effective in patients in whom PDT cannot be used, such as those with minimal classic choroidal neovascularization (CNV) or pigment epithelial detachment. In some small reports, a combination of PDT with triamcinolone acetate injection has been reported to be beneficial in the treatment occult CNVs with pigment epithelial detachment, with a lower risk of pigment epithelial tears.
- Further studies are investigating whether combination treatment with PDT and intravitreal administration of antiangiogenetic drugs might have a synergistic effect. It might also be possible that a combination of drugs with different effects (e.g., VEGF antagonist and corticosteroids) could have a synergistic effect.
- Treatment schedules have been defined for several drugs, but with the exception of severe disease progression, it has not yet been clarified when it is safe to stop drug administration. A beneficial effect of drug administration over 2 years has been reported in some studies.
- Neither the impact of reduced visual loss in neovascular AMD nor the effect on health-care costs can be calculated at the moment for any of the drugs.
- In addition to CNV treatment, some drugs may also be effective in the treatment of diabetic macular edema.

Fluorescein Angiography

- Fluorescein angiography is a major tool for following up the success of treatment after intravitreal drug administration.
- Specific changes have not been demonstrated after drug administration. A reduction in the size of the lesion and a reduction in the associated hyperfluorescence due to reduced leakage can be observed. Staining will be present in fibrotic tissue.
- It has yet to be established how often fluorescein angiography or optic coherence tomography should be carried out during treatment with drugs that have to be injected frequently.

References

Cunningham ET Jr, Adamis AP, Altaweel M, et al. A phase II randomized double-masked trial of pegaptanib, an anti-vascular endothelial growth factor aptamer, for diabetic macular edema. Ophthalmology 2005;112:1747–57.

D'Amico DJ, Goldberg MF, Hudson H, et al. Anecortave acetate as monotherapy for treatment of subfoveal neovascularization in age-related macular degeneration: twelve-month clinical outcomes. Ophthalmology 2003;110:2372–83.

Gragoudas ES, Adamis AP, Cunningham ET Jr, et al. Pegaptanib for neovascular age-related macular degeneration. N Engl J Med 2004;351:2805–16.

Heier JS, Antoszyk AN, Pavan PR, et al: Ranibizumab for treatment of neovascular age-related macular degeneration a phase I/II multicenter, controlled, multidose study. Ophthalmology 2006 (epub ahead of print).

Husain D, Kim I, Gauthier D, et al. Safety and efficacy of intravitreal injection of ranibizumab in combination with verteporfin PDT on experimental choroidal neovascularization in the monkey. Arch Ophthalmol 2005;123:509–16.

Michels S, Rosenfeld PJ, Puliafito CA, et al. Systemic bevacizumab (Avastin) therapy for neovascular age-related macular degeneration: twelve-week results of an uncontrolled open-label clinical study. Ophthalmology 2005;112:1035–47.

Pauleikhoff D, Bornfeld N, Gabel VP, et al. [The position of the Retinological Society, the German Ophthalmological Society and the Professional Association of Ophthalmologists: comments on the current therapy for neovascular AMD; in German.] Klin Monatsbl Augenheilkd 2005;222:381–8.

Schmidt-Erfurth U, Michels S, Michels R, Aue A. Anecortave acetate for the treatment of subfoveal choroidal neovascularization secondary to age-related macular degeneration. Eur J Ophthalmol 2005;15:482–5.

Van de Moere A, Sandhu SS, Kak R, Mitchell KW, Talks SJ. Effect of posterior juxtascleral triamcinolone acetonide on choroidal neovascular growth after photodynamic therapy with verteporfin. Ophthalmology 2005;112:1896–903.

3

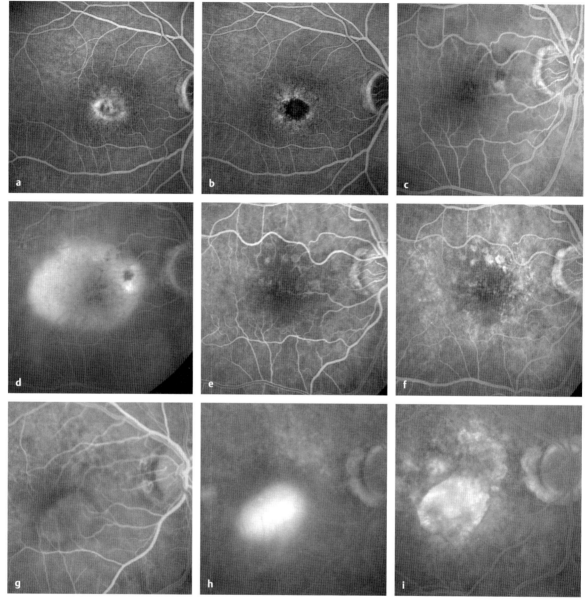

Fig. 3.14a–i Angiography after intravitreal drug administration for choroidal neovascularization

a Late phase. Before treatment, an area of subfoveal choroidal neovascularization with moderate leakage is present.

b Late phase. Six weeks after one injection of pegaptanib (Macugen), the choroidal neovascularization is barely detectable.

c Arteriovenous phase (in a different patient). Retinal angiomatous proliferation with a small hemorrhage before treatment.

d Late phase. Marked leakage delineates an associated retinal pigment epithelial detachment.

e Arteriovenous phase. Six months after photodynamic therapy and intravitreal injection of triamcinolone acetate (4 mg), marked regression of the lesion has occurred.

f Late phase. Small window defects can be seen superior to the fovea. No leakage and no retinal pigment epithelial detachment remains. The patient's visual acuity increased from 0.2 to 0.5.

g Arteriovenous phase (in a different patient). Classic subfoveal choroidal neovascularization before treatment.

h Late phase. Marked leakage from the choroidal neovascularization.

i Late phase. Seven months after one session of photodynamic therapy (PDT) and intravitreal injection of triamcinolone acetate (4 mg), the lesion shows staining, without leakage. No additional PDT has so far been necessary.

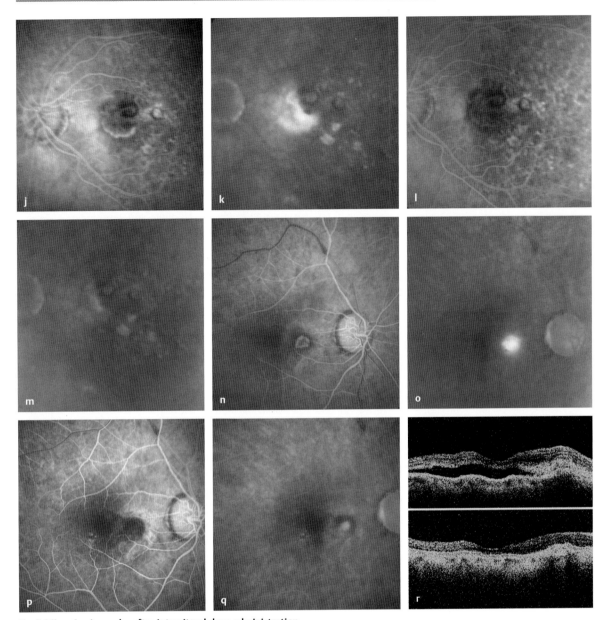

Fig. 3.14j–r Angiography after intravitreal drug administration for choroidal neovascularization

j   Arteriovenous phase (different patient). A predominantely classic choroidal neovascularisation is delineated with a neovascular network.

k   Late phase. Marked leakage extends beyond the borders of the lesion in the arteriovenous phase.

l   Arteriovenous phase 4 weeks after intravitreal bevacizumab (Avastin) injection. The neovascular network is visible with less perfusion.

m Late phase. The lesion shows staining without obvious leakage.

n   Early arteriovenous phase (different patient). An extrafoveal classic choroidal neovascularisation presents between fovea and optic disc.

o   Late phase. Marked leakage extends beyond the borders of the lesion in the early phase.

p   Early arteriovenous phase 12 weeks after intravitreal bevacizumab (Avastin) injection in combination with photodynamic therapy. Hypofluorescence is present in the region of the previous choroidal neovascularisation, with slight surrounding hyperfluorescence. The neovascular network is visible with less perfusion.

q   Late phase. The lesion shows staining without obvious leakage.

r   Optic coherence tomography: Upper image corrsponds to **n** and **o**, prior to treatment subretinal fluid and retinal edema are present. Lower image corresponds to **p** and **q** with regressed subretinal fluid and retinal edema.

4.1 Retinitis Pigmentosa   *Ulrich Kellner*

Epidemiology, Pathophysiology, and Clinical Presentation

- Retinitis pigmentosa is the most common group of retinal dystrophies (with a prevalence of approximately one in 5000).
- Mutations in at least 32 genes have been associated with the development of nonsyndromic retinitis pigmentosa. It can be expected that additional gene associations will be discovered.
- The products of these genes are either expressed in the retinal pigment epithelium (RPE) or the photoreceptors. Within the photoreceptor–retinal pigment epithelium complex, the degeneration of one cell type is followed by the degeneration of the others. It is not possible to recognize clinically in this process whether the primary damage is located in the photoreceptor or in the RPE. It is usually the rods that are mainly affected, but degeneration of the rods subsequently leads to degeneration of the cones.
- All patterns of inheritance can occur (autosomal-dominant, autosomal-recessive, X-linked, mitochondrial). In some syndromes, combinations with disorders in other organs are not uncommon (e. g., with hearing impairment in Usher's syndrome).
- The time of onset ranges from congenital conditions (as in Leber congenital amaurosis) to courses with very minor abnormalities that may only be identified accidentally in later life. Due to this variability, it is very difficult to assess the prognosis in individual cases.
- Clinically, the course of the disease is characterized by the onset of impaired night vision. Slowly progressive loss of peripheral visual fields develops, often leaving only an isolated central visual field intact. Electroretinography (ERG) may show severely reduced responses or an absence of detectable responses.

Fluorescein Angiography

- Fluorescein angiography is not necessary for the diagnosis of retinitis pigmentosa.
- Loss of the choriocapillaris and defects in the RPE are already recognizable in the early phase.
- In the late phase, leakage can be observed when cystoid macular edema or vascular abnormalities similar to those in Coats disease are present.

Fundus Autofluorescence

- A reduction in or absence of fundus autofluorescence indicates areas with loss of photoreceptors and/or of the RPE.
- A ring of increased perifoveal autofluorescence can be observed in some patients. This corresponds to the border of central retinal function. Concentric progression of the ring can be observed over time.
- The fovea can show normal, increased, or reduced autofluorescence.

- Further research is needed in order to define the prognostic value of fundus autofluorescence imaging.

Diagnosis and Treatment

- The initial diagnosis of retinitis pigmentosa is based on perimetry, ophthalmoscopy in mydriasis, and an ERG.
- Even if typical ophthalmoscopic findings are present, at least one ERG recording is recommended, as there may be significant discrepancies between the morphological and functional findings and assessment of retinal function provides the best basis for counseling the patient.
- Fundus autofluorescence may detect morphological alterations that are not visible with ophthalmoscopy.
- Fluorescein angiography is only indicated in the presence of abnormal Coats-like vessels or when cystoid macular edema is suspected. The latter can also be diagnosed with optical coherence tomography. This can be particularly recommended, as severe cystoid macular edema may resemble macular hole formation.
- Cystoid macular edema may respond well to oral acetazolamide administration.
- Photocoagulation limits the progression of abnormal vessel formation in the few patients with Coats-like vessels.
- There are as yet no means of treating the condition, although clinical trials of gene therapy are being prepared.
- Refractive errors should be corrected and, where applicable, the use of special filter glasses and low-vision aids can be very helpful.
- Nutritional supplements (e. g., vitamin A palmitate, docosahexaenoic acid) may delay the progression of some forms of retinitis pigmentosa.
- Early cataract formation is frequent and requires surgery, as subcapsular cataracts typically develop on the posterior pole of the lens, directly in front of the remainder of the central visual field.

References

Gass JD. Retinitis pigmentosa (rod-cone dystrophies). In: Gass JD, ed. Stereoscopic atlas of macular diseases: diagnosis and treatment, 4th ed. St. Louis: Mosby, 1997: 352–8.

Rivolta C, Sharon D, DeAngelis MM, Dryja TP. Retinitis pigmentosa and allied diseases: numerous diseases, genes, and inheritance patterns. Hum Mol Genet 2002;11:1219–27.

Robson AG, Egan CA, Luong VA, et al. Comparison of fundus autofluorescence with photopic and scotopic fine-matrix mapping in patients with retinitis pigmentosa and normal visual acuity. Invest Ophthalmol Vis Sci 2004;45:4119–25

Weleber RG, Gregory-Evans K. Retinitis pigmentosa and allied disorders. In: Ryan SJ, ed. Retina, 4th ed. Philadelphia: Elsevier, 2006:395–498.

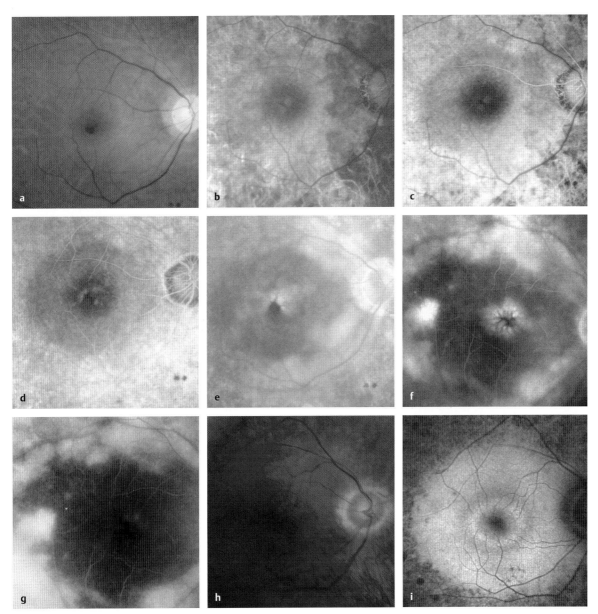

Fig. 4.1a–i Retinitis pigmentosa

a Color photograph. Constricted vessels, peripheral choriocapillaris atrophy, and a cystoid macular edema that almost has the appearance of a macular hole.

b Early phase. Large choroidal vessels are visible in the area of the choriocapillaris atrophy.

c Late early phase. An oval area with a relatively conserved retinal pigment epithelium can be seen at the posterior pole.

d Early late phase. Initial perifoveal leakage.

e Late phase. Cystoid macular edema and choroidal hyperfluorescence in the peripheral areas, with choriocapillary and retinal pigment epithelial loss.

f Late phase (in a different patient). Cystoid macular edema.

g Late phase (in the same patient as in **f**). Reduction in the cystoid macular edema after oral acetazolamide therapy.

h Color photograph. Unobtrusive pigment epithelium irregularities at the posterior pole.

i Fundus autofluorescence. Peripheral destruction of the retinal pigment epithelium and a pericentral ring of increased autofluorescence.

4.2 Choroideremia and Gyrate Atrophy   *Ulrich Kellner*

Choroideremia

Epidemiology, Pathophysiology, and Clinical Presentation

- An X-linked condition, choroideremia is a generalized form of choroidal dystrophy that starts in the mid-periphery of the retina and is associated with mutations in the *CHM* (*REP-1*) gene.
- As in retinitis pigmentosa, symptoms start with night blindness and mid-peripheral visual field loss with progressive concentric narrowing, whereas visual acuity and color vision remain very good for a longer period of time.
- In males, fine pigment-epithelial irregularities can be observed initially, followed by small mid-peripheral areas of choroidal atrophy with fuzzy edges, which later converge. A central island of intact choroid often persists for a longer period at the posterior pole. The retinal vessels usually change very little.
- In female carriers, distinct pigment changes are almost always present over the whole retina. Retinal function is generally normal. Symptomatic female carriers with a disease progression similar to that in males are rare.

Fluorescein Angiography

- Fluorescein angiography allows early detection of affected choroidal areas.
- As in the clinical findings, choriocapillaris atrophy with fuzzy edges can be seen with angiography. The borders of atrophic areas are lined with increased fluorescence in the late phase.

Fundus Autofluorescence

- Fundus autofluorescence can identify areas of retinal pigment epithelial loss in males.
- In females, fundus autofluorescence shows a speckled pattern, with small areas of reduced autofluorescence. This autofluorescence pattern may suggest carrier status as an incidental finding in women who do not have a family history of the condition.

Diagnosis and Treatment

- In men with the early stages of choroideremia, with alterations in the retinal pigment epithelium, it is possible for the condition to be confused with retinitis pigmentosa.
- More serious, however, and more burdensome for the patients affected, is misdiagnosis of this condition as retinitis pigmentosa, on the basis of the changes in the retina, in female carriers—since these patients do not generally experience any relevant functional disturbances. Fundus autofluorescence is recommended for differential diagnosis.

- Full-field electroretinography (ERG) shows that in men, rod-dependent responses are more reduced than cone-dependent ones. In women, the ERG is generally normal. In contrast, the fundus is usually normal in female carriers of X-linked retinitis pigmentosa, but the amplitudes of the ERG are more often reduced in these cases.
- Molecular-genetic diagnosis is possible, but this is complex and is not necessary in clear-cut cases.
- There are no causal treatments.
- It is important to exclude gyrate atrophy, a less frequent condition, during differential diagnosis.

Gyrate Atrophy

Epidemiology, Pathophysiology, and Clinical Presentation

- Gyrate atrophy is an autosomal-recessive condition involving generalized choroidal dystrophy that starts in the mid-periphery of the retina and is associated with mutations in the ornithine aminotransferase gene (*OAT*).
- In contrast to choroideremia, the borders of the atrophic areas are sharply delineated.
- Otherwise, the clinical course is similar to that in choroideremia, with confluence of patchy choroidal atrophy and progression to the posterior pole. In addition, early cataract formation is observed.

Fluorescein Angiography

- Fluorescein angiography reveals choriocapillaris atrophy, with sharply delineated edges and increased fluorescence on the border of the lesions.

Diagnosis and Treatment

- The ERG shows that rod-dependent responses are more reduced than cone-dependent ones.
- Molecular-genetic diagnosis is possible, but is not necessary in clear-cut cases.
- Markedly elevated ornithine blood levels are pathognomonic.
- A specific diet may influence the course of the disease.

References

Do DV, Zhang K, Garabaldi DC, Carr RE, Sunness JS. Hereditary choroidal disease. In: Ryan SJ, ed. Retina, 4th ed. Philadelphia, Elsevier, 2006:499–508.

Gass JD. Atypical forms of retinitis pigmentosa. In: Gass JD, ed. Stereoscopic atlas of macular diseases: diagnosis and treatment, 4th ed. St. Louis: Mosby, 1997:358–81.

Kaiser-Kupfer MI, Caruso RC, Valle D, Reed GF. Use of an arginine-restricted diet to slow progression of visual loss in patients with gyrate atrophy. Arch Ophthalmol 2004;122:982–4.

Roberts MF, Fishman GA, Roberts DK, et al. Retrospective, longitudinal, and cross sectional study of visual acuity impairment in choroideraemia. Br J Ophthalmol 2002;86:658–62.

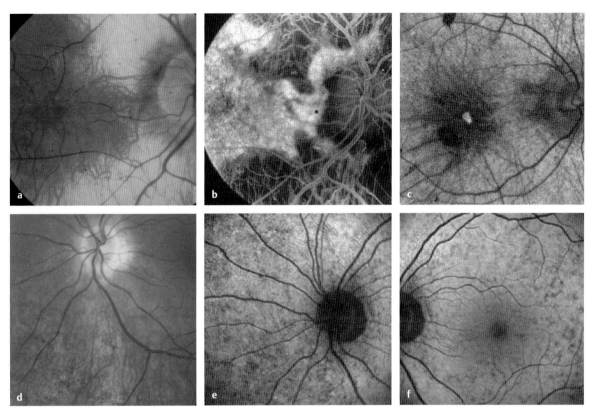

Fig. 4.2a–f Choroideremia

a Color photograph. Temporal and subfoveal to the disk, a patch of choriocapillaris is still present; more peripherally, only a few large choroidal vessels can be detected.

b Arteriovenous phase. Only a few large choroidal vessels are visible in the atrophic areas; retained choriocapillaris and pigment epithelium with pigment epithelium defects can be seen at the posterior pole and temporal to the optic disc.

c Fundus autofluorescence (in a different patient). A small island of retained pigment epithelium is detectable through a patch of remaining autofluorescence.

d Color photograph in a female carrier. Several variably distinct pigmentations can be seen, while visual acuity, color vision, the field of vision, and electroretinography were normal.

e Fundus autofluorescence. A speckled pattern with small areas of reduced or increased autofluorescence is visible nasally.

f Fundus autofluorescence. At the posterior pole, there is a speckled pattern with small areas of reduced autofluorescence.

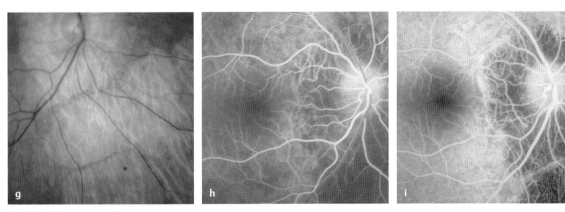

Fig. 4.2g–i Gyrate atrophy

g Color photograph. Sharply delineated peripapillary choroid atrophy, which continues toward the periphery below the optic disc.

h Early phase. Only the large choroidal vessels are visible in the affected areas.

i Arteriovenous phase. A small bridge of retained choriocapillaris is recognizable below the optic disc. The choroid outside the affected areas appears to be intact.

4.3 X-Linked Congenital Retinoschisis   *Ulrich Kellner*

Epidemiology, Pathophysiology, and Clinical Presentation

- X-linked retinoschisis is a frequent form of retinal dystrophy in young males associated with mutations in the *RS1* gene. The *RS1* gene product is important for cell-to-cell interaction in the retina.
- The morphological changes vary from severe retinoschisis affecting the complete retina at 3 months of age to unobtrusive foveal alterations that are not infrequently overlooked during ophthalmoscopic examinations.
- Clinically, diminished but generally stable visual acuity of approximately 0.2 is evident. Hyperopia is common.
- Ophthalmoscopically, changes can always be found in the macula, often as a star-shaped retinoschisis. Peripheral retinoschisis may be found in fewer than half of the cases, most often in the temporal inferior quadrant. Peripheral retinoschisis extends to the center only rarely.
- In the retinoschisis region, the inner layer of the retina may disintegrate between the retinal vessels, so that free retinal vessels can be seen in the vitreous body. Vitreous hemorrhage can arise from these vessels. Retinal detachment can result if breaks in the outer layer develop in addition to disintegration of the inner layer.
- Generally, complications such as retinal detachments and vitreous hemorrhage are rare and appear more often in the first decade of life.
- In later life, the central retinoschisis regresses, and often only central pigment mottling is visible. Slowly progressive deterioration in visual acuity occurs in old age.

Fluorescein Angiography and Fundus Autofluorescence

- Fluorescein angiography is generally not required.
- Occasionally, folds in the inner retina can be observed with angiography, but the examination may also be completely normal.
- Autofluorescence may show foveal abnormalities, most likely due to altered passage of the exciting and emitted light in the schisis folds.

Diagnosis and Treatment

- The diagnosis is easily made when an obvious foveal retinoschisis is present.
- Discrete central retinoschisis can be detected with optical coherence tomography.
- Full-field electroretinography (ERG) often shows a "negative ERG," with predominantly reduced b-wave amplitudes. However, some cases without a negative ERG have been reported. In young male patients who do not have ophthalmoscopically clear retinoschisis and with a negative ERG, X-linked congenital stationary night blindness must be included in the differential diagnosis.
- Molecular-genetic diagnosis with *RS1* gene analysis is advisable when providing family counseling.
- There are no causal treatments. Various types of visual aids (e. g., magnifying glasses) can be prescribed as needed.
- Prophylactic laser coagulation on the edge of the retinoschisis should be strictly avoided, since this is linked to a higher risk of retinal detachment. In vitreous hemorrhage, spontaneous remission usually occurs. Surgical procedures are required in retinal detachment, but the chances of success are limited.
- Symptomatic female carriers of X-linked retinoschisis have not been observed. Familial retinoschisis also affecting females is extremely rare.

References

Apushkin MA, Fishman GA, Rajagopalan AS. Fundus findings and longitudinal study of visual acuity loss in patients with x-linked retinoschisis. Retina 2005;25:612–8.

Bradshaw K, George N, Moore A, Trump D, Mutations of the *XLRS1* gene cause abnormalities of the photoreceptor as well as inner retinal responses of the ERG. Doc Ophthalmol 1999;98:153–73.

Edwards AO, Robertson Jr. JE. Hereditary vitreoretinal degenerations. In: Ryan SJ. ed. Retina, 4th ed. Philadelphia, Elsevier, 2006:519–38.

Tantri A, Vrabec TR, Cu-Unjieng A, et al. X-linked retinoschisis: a clinical and molecular genetic review. Surv Ophthalmol 2004;49:214–30.

Weber BHF, Kellner U. X-linked retinoschisis. Hum Mol Genet [in press].

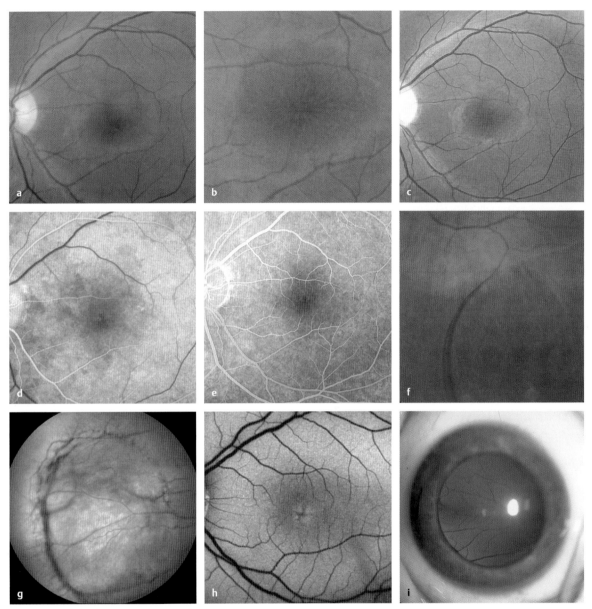

Fig. 4.3a–i X-linked Congenital retinoschisis

a Color photograph. The central retinoschisis is barely recognizable in this overview.

b Color photograph. The enlargement makes the central folds clearly visible.

c Black-and-white image. The changes in the fovea are also clearly visible.

d Early phase. Unobtrusive foveal hyperfluorescence.

e Arteriovenous phase. Unchanged unobtrusive foveal hyperfluorescence.

f Color photograph (in a different patient). There is peripheral retinoschisis, indicated by the shadow on the outer retinal layer of the elevated vessel.

g Infrared imaging (in a different patient). Peripheral retinoschisis without extension to the ora is visible in this wide-field image.

h Fundus autofluorescence (left eye of the patient in **g**). Central irregularities in the autofluorescence due to foveal retinoschisis.

i Color photograph (in a different patient). Severe retinoschisis in a 5-month-old infant, with an upper and lower schisis bulla, leaving only a central slit for viewing from the undetached posterior pole. The fellow eye had a similar retinoschisis.

4.4 Stargardt Disease   *Ulrich Kellner*

Epidemiology, Pathophysiology, and Clinical Presentation

- Stargardt disease is the most common type of macular dystrophy. The form with autosomal-recessive inheritance is associated with mutations in the *ABCA4* gene. The *ABCA4* gene product is a transport protein that allows transport of vitamin A derivatives from the photoreceptor to the retinal pigment epithelium. Similar fundus abnormalities with autosomal-dominant inheritance are extremely rare.
- Stargardt disease is usually regarded as a form of macular dystrophy. Recent molecular-genetic research has shown that cone–rod dystrophy with autosomal-recessive inheritance is frequently associated with mutations in the *ABCA4* gene. There is a continuous spectrum of clinical expression, ranging from Stargardt disease limited to the macula to severe cone–rod dystrophy with progression to blindness, with no definite distinction between the two forms.
- Several clinical classifications of Stargardt disease have been published; these tend to reflect the variability in the development of the dystrophy rather than typical stages of disease progression.
- The disease becomes symptomatic most commonly in the first two decades of life, but can also become manifest later.
- The initial symptoms are an acute reduction in visual acuity, in which the background of the eye can still appear completely normal. At this stage, multifocal electroretinography already shows abnormalities.
- After a decrease in visual acuity to about 0.1, stabilization with only minor further progression is often encountered.
- Ophthalmoscopically, variable distinct yellow flecks (fundus flavimaculatus) and central pigment epithelium defects ranging up to bull's-eye maculopathy can be seen.
- In the late stages, choroidal neovascularization (CNV) sometimes develops.

Fluorescein Angiography

- In Stargardt disease, angiography often reveals a blockage of the background fluorescence ("dark choroid"). Since the advent of molecular-genetic analysis, it has been possible to show that dark choroid is not present in all eyes with Stargardt disease. Fluorescein angiography is therefore no longer necessary for the diagnosis of Stargardt disease.
- The yellow flecks may show amplified or reduced fluorescence; in addition, pigment epithelium defects may be present in a variety of forms.

Fundus Autofluorescence

- Fundus autofluorescence has replaced fluorescein angiography in Stargardt disease.
- The flecks may show either increased or reduced autofluorescence, and pigment epithelial atrophy is indicated by an absence of autofluorescence.
- There is wide variability in the autofluorescence findings; whether they have any predictive value has yet to be determined.

Diagnosis and Treatment

- The diagnosis is quite easy to reach in cases of typical fundus changes. In the early stage, if the morphology is still normal, testing of visual acuity, color vision, and the central visual field may indicate abnormalities, and multifocal electroretinography can objectively detect central retinal dysfunction.
- In the late stages, if there is distinct atrophy and regression of yellow flecks, it is not possible not distinguish the condition from the atrophic late phase of other forms of macular degeneration.
- Fluorescein angiography can detect the development of CNVs. In the presence of CNV treatment similar to that in the established regimens in age-related macular degeneration is recommended.
- A molecular-genetic diagnosis is possible by analyzing the *ABCA4* gene.
- There is no causal treatment; low-vision aids can be prescribed, depending on function.
- Vitamin A supplementation is not recommended.

References

Koenekoop RK. The gene for Stargardt disease, *ABCA4*, is a major retinal gene: a mini-review. Ophthalmic Genet 2003;24:75–80.

Klevering BJ, Deutmann AF, Maugeri A, Cremers FP, Hoyng CB. The spectrum of retinal phenotypes caused by mutations in the *ABCA4* gene. Graefes Arch Clin Exp Ophthalmol 2005;243:90–100.

Lois N, Halfyard AS, Bird AC, et al. Fundus autofluorescence in Stargardt macular dystrophy–fundus flavimaculatus. Am J Ophthalmol 2004;138:55–63.

Oh KT, Weleber RG, Stone EM, Oh DM, Rosenow J, Billinslea AM. Electroretinographic findings in patients with Stargardt disease and fundus flavimaculatus. Retina 2004;24:920–8.

Rotenstreich Y, Fishman GA, Anderson RJ. Visual acuity loss and clinical observations in a large series of patients with Stargardt disease. Ophthalmology 2003;110:1151–8.

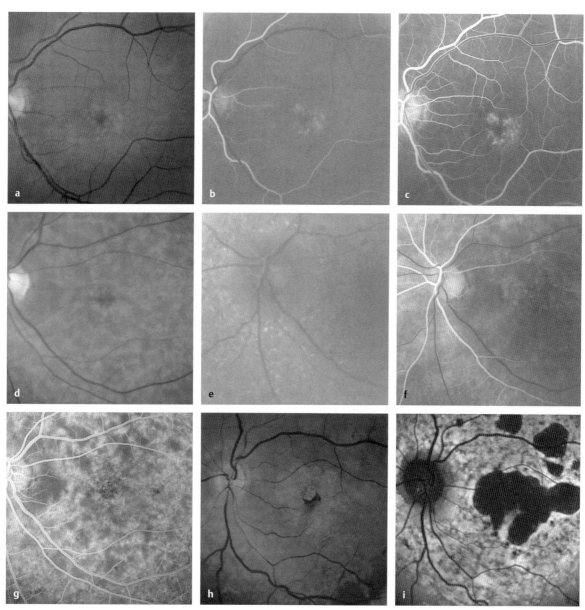

Fig. 4.**4a–i Stargardt disease**

a Color photograph. Central yellow flecks and pigment epithelium defects.

b Early phase. Reduced choroidal fluorescence and central pigment epithelium defects.

c Early arteriovenous phase. Continued low-level choroidal fluorescence and unchanged central pigment epithelium defects.

d Color photograph. Distinct fundus flavimaculatus.

e Early phase. At the start of retinal filling, a few flecks show autofluorescence.

f Late early phase. The flecks are no longer recognizable.

g Late phase. Distinct coloring of the flavimaculatus flecks and the pigment epithelium defects.

h Color photograph. Central chorioatrophic area and fundus flavimaculatus.

i Fundus autofluorescence. Absent autofluorescence in the chorioatrophic lesion and augmented fluorescence in the flecks.

4.5 Best Disease (Vitelliform Macular Dystrophy) *Ulrich Kellner*

Epidemiology, Pathophysiology, and Clinical Presentation

- Best disease is a form of macular dystrophy with autosomal-dominant inheritance, associated with mutations in the *VMD2* gene. The *VMD2* gene product plays a role in ion transport membrane channels on the basal membrane of the retinal pigment epithelium cells.
- The diagnosis of Best disease is generally easy, owing to its characteristic ophthalmoscopic image.
- Due to reduced penetrance, some carriers of the mutation in an affected family may remain without clinically recognizable alterations; individual cases of Best disease without family case histories can also occur.
- The onset is often in the first two decades of life, but later manifestations can occur up to the 6th decade of life.
- Histologically, an increasing accumulation of lipofuscin-like material in the retinal pigment epithelium is seen, where syncytia from pigment epithelium cells can arise that match the clinical image.
- Ophthalmoscopically, an elevated central yellow lesion larger than one disk diameter is generally visible initially. Lesions that do not affect the center and multifocal lesions are less frequent.
- Later, pseudohypopyon may develop, showing a horizontal level of yellow material, which is then followed by extensive loss of the yellow material.
- In the late stage only a chorioatrophic lesion without yellow material remains. Choroidal neovascularization (CNV) has been observed, as well as pigmentations similar to pattern dystrophies.

Fluorescein Angiography

- Fluorescein angiography is not essential for the diagnosis, but should be considered when there is a suspicion of choroidal neovascularization.
- The lipofuscin in the vitelliform lesion blocks the background fluorescence. These areas appear hypofluorescent during the entire course of the angiogram.
- If a reduction in the lipofuscin takes place, loss of the retinal pigment epithelium also occurs in these areas, and hyperfluorescence is consequently expected.
- Lesions that retain both portions show a mixed image.

- In the late stage, only an atrophic zone with hyperfluorescence is still recognizable.

Fundus Autofluorescence

- Vitelliform lesions present with increased autofluorescence; areas with atrophy show reduced autofluorescence.
- In the late stages, fundus autofluorescence may detect small areas of increased autofluorescence, indicating remnants of vitelliform material.

Diagnosis and Treatment

- As a rule, the diagnosis is carried out with ophthalmoscopy. In distinct central vitelliform lesions, visual acuity can be normal, but a reduction in visual acuity (to about 0.1) should be expected over time.
- The diagnosis can be confirmed by an absent or notably reduced light rise (Arden ratio) in an electrooculogram (EOG). This is also seen in clinically inconspicuous carriers of the gene mutation. However, in few cases the EOG is normal in Best disease.
- Best disease can be confirmed by the detection of mutations in the *VMD2* gene. This is worthwhile in individual cases and for counseling of clinical healthy family members.
- There is no causal treatment. In patients with a loss of visual acuity, it is important to prescribe low-vision aids.
- Fluorescein angiography can detect the development of CNVs. In the presence of CNV treatment similar to that in the established regimens in age-related macular degeneration is recommended.

References

Deutman AF, Hoyng CB, van Lith-Verhoeven JJC. Macular dystrophies. In: Ryan SJ, ed. Retina, 4th ed. Philadelphia, Elsevier, 2006: 1163–210.

Gass JD. Best's disease. In: Gass JD, ed. Stereoscopic atlas of macular diseases: diagnosis and treatment, 4th ed. St. Louis: Mosby, 1997: 304–11.

Renner AB, Tillack H, Kraus H, et al. Late onset is common in Best macular dystrophy associated with *VMD2* gene mutation. Ophthalmology 2005;112:586–92.

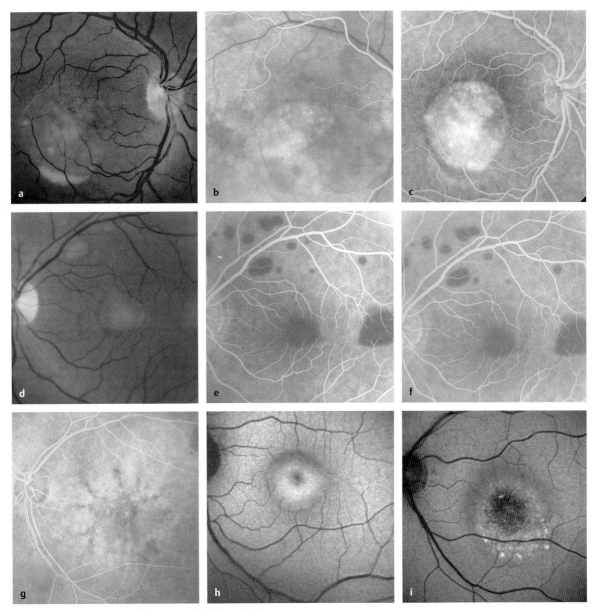

Fig. 4.5a–i Best disease (vitelliform macular dystrophy)

a Color photograph. Advanced stage of vitelliform macular dystrophy, with extensive deterioration of the yellow material.

b Early phase. Window defects are recognizable in the region of the lesion.

c Late phase. Clear window defects without leakage in the area of the clinically visible lesion. This image remains basically unchanged during angiography.

d Color photograph. Multiple vitelliform lesions.

e Arteriovenous phase. Blockage of the background fluorescence in all vitelliform lesions.

f Late phase. Persistent blockage caused by the vitelliform lesions.

g Arteriovenous phase (in a different patient). Late stage of Best disease: central window defects with a faint radiating pattern.

h Fundus autofluorescence. Vitelliform stage: decidedly increased fluorescence in the vitelliform lesion.

i Fundus autofluorescence. Atrophic late stage: increased autofluorescence can only be seen in a few areas; in other areas, the atrophy of the retinal pigment epithelium shows correspondingly reduced autofluorescence.

4.6 Adult Vitelliform Macular Dystrophy and Pattern Dystrophies   *Ulrich Kellner*

Adult Vitelliform Macular Dystrophy

Epidemiology, Pathophysiology, and Clinical Presentation

- Adult vitelliform macular dystrophy (AVMD) is probably the most common form of macular dystrophy in adults, becoming symptomatic between the 3rd and 5th decades of life. Various diseases with similar clinical appearances are most probably also summarized under this heading.
- AVMD often appears in sporadic cases, although autosomal-dominant inheritance has been described. The expression is very variable.
- In individual cases of AVMD, mutations in the peripherin/*RDS* gene or *VMD2* gene have been described, emphasizing the heterogeneous composition of the group.
- In contrast to other forms of inherited macular dystrophy, progression in AVMD often differs between the two eyes, so that good visual acuity may be maintained in at least one eye.
- Ophthalmoscopically, a yellow lesion (smaller than one optic disc diameter) is usually found in both eyes (in contrast to the larger lesions in Best disease), sometimes with pigmentation within the lesion.
- Choroidal neovascularization may develop in some cases.

Fluorescein Angiography

- Fluorescein angiography in many cases shows a dark center surrounded by a ring of hyperfluorescence. The angiographic findings may be nearly normal or show nonspecific hyperfluorescence in about 40% of cases.

Fundus Autofluorescence

- A distinct spot of increased autofluorescence can be detected with fundus autofluorescence in about four out of five cases.

Diagnosis and Treatment

- The diagnosis is based on the ophthalmoscopic findings and supported by alterations seen on angiography and fundus autofluorescence.
- Molecular-genetic analysis is of limited value at present.
- There is no causal treatment. Low-vision aids should be used if applicable.
- Fluorescein angiography can detect the development of CNVs. In the presence of CNV treatment similar to that in the established regimens in age-related macular degeneration is recommended.

Pattern Dystrophies

Epidemiology, Pathophysiology, and Clinical Presentation

- Pattern dystrophies are another heterogeneous group of macular dystrophies, although less frequent. Sporadic cases and autosomal-dominant inheritance have been observed.
- In individual cases, mutations in the peripherin/*RDS* gene have been described.
- Pattern dystrophies show changes in the retinal pigment epithelium in a pattern arrangement that usually has a less marked ophthalmoscopic appearance than in fluorescein angiography or on fundus autofluorescence.
- Choroidal neovascularization may develop in some cases.

Fluorescein Angiography and Fundus Autofluorescence

- Fluorescein angiography is very useful for identifying pigment epithelium changes in pattern dystrophies, but autofluorescence also shows pigment epithelium changes and is therefore generally sufficient.

Diagnosis and Treatment

- The diagnosis is based on the clinical findings and in particular on the angiographic and fundus autofluorescence findings.
- Molecular-genetic analysis is of limited value at present.
- There is no causal treatment. Low-vision aids should be used if applicable.
- Fluorescein angiography can detect the development of CNVs. In the presence of CNV treatment similar to that in the established regimens in age-related macular degeneration is recommended.

References

Battaglia Parodi M, Da Pozzo S, Ravalico G. Photodynamic therapy for choroidal neovascularization associated with pattern dystrophy. Retina 2003;23:171–6.

Deutman AF, Hoyng CB, van Lith-Verhoeven JJC. Macular dystrophies. In: Ryan SJ, ed. Retina, 4th ed. Philadelphia, Elsevier, 2006: 1163–210.

Gass JD. Autosomal dominant pattern dystrophies of the RPE. In: Gass JD, ed. Stereoscopic atlas of macular diseases: diagnosis and treatment, 4th ed. St. Louis: Mosby, 1997: 314–25.

Renner AB, Tillack H, Kraus H, et al. Morphology and functional characteristics in adult vitelliform macular dystrophy. Retina 2004;24:929–39.

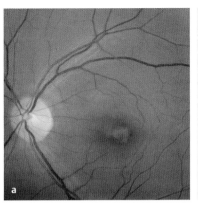

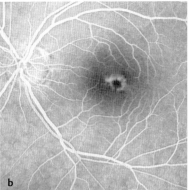

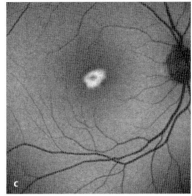

Fig. 4.6a–c Adult vitelliform macular dystrophy

a Color photograph. Central yellow lesion < 1 optic disc diameter. Pigmentation is recognizable in the lesion.

b Arteriovenous phase. Central blockage with ambient hyperfluorescence, which remains constant during the course of the angiogram.

c Fundus autofluorescence (different patient): Increased autofluorescence with central blockage due to a pigmented area can be seen in the lesion.

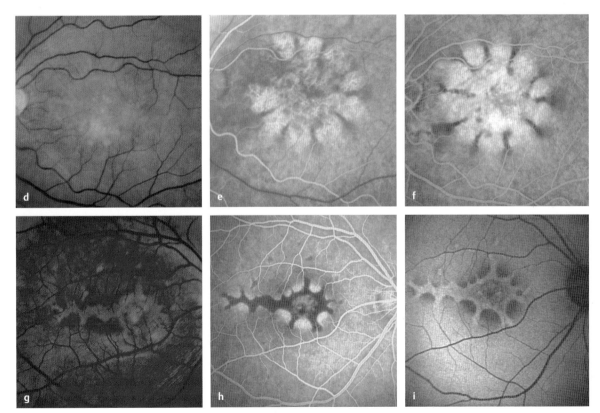

Fig. 4.6d–i Pattern dystrophy

d Color photograph. Pigment epithelial defects without a clear pattern on the posterior pole.

e Early phase. Easily recognizable pattern, with hypofluorescent and hyperfluorescent areas.

f Late phase. Unchanged display of the pattern.

g Color photograph. Pigment epithelial defects with a recognizable pattern in a case of pattern dystrophy.

h Arteriovenous phase. The pattern corresponds to the ophthalmoscopically visible lesion.

i Fundus autofluorescence. A similarly good depiction of the pattern. The blockage in the angiogram is related to increased autofluorescence (increased lipofuscin).

4.7 Hydroxychloroquine and Chloroquine Retinopathy   *Ulrich Kellner*

Epidemiology, Pathophysiology, and Clinical Presentation

- There is only a risk of hydroxychloroquine or chloroquine retinopathy after long-term administration, not after short-term treatment—e. g., for prophylaxis against malaria.
- Long-term treatment with hydroxychloroquine and chloroquine is given in various autoimmune diseases (e. g., lupus erythematosus and rheumatic diseases).
- Hydroxychloroquine treatment is preferable to chloroquine, as hydroxychloroquine has less ocular toxicity. It is not possible to define an absolutely safe daily dosage or a total quantity for either chloroquine or hydroxychloroquine.
- Hydroxychloroquine and chloroquine have a high affinity with melanin and are deposited in the retinal pigment epithelium. However, animal experiments have shown that the first changes (with storage of small inclusion bodies) take place in the ganglion cells and later in all retinal cells. Up to a specific point, the inclusion bodies can resolve completely after discontinuation of chloroquine intake. The toxic damage is initiated by the degeneration of the photoreceptors, with subsequent degeneration of other retinal cells and the retinal pigment epithelium.
- For reasons that are not understood, the foveal cones remain intact for a long period, so that clinically pericentral scotoma can lead to reading difficulties when single-letter visual acuity is still good. In addition, patients may experience color vision defects. Decreasing visual acuity and loss of visual field are observed if the medication is not discontinued.

Fluorescein Angiography

- With fluorescein angiography, verifiable changes in the retinal pigment epithelium generally develop after retinal dysfunction becomes apparent.
- Fluorescein angiography can be used as an additional procedure, particularly in patients in whom other examinations have produced unclear results.
- Perifoveal window defects in the retinal pigment epithelium appear either as a full oval (as in bull's-eye maculopathy), or only as an open oval. Leakages are not encountered.
- Peripheral pigment epithelial alterations only occur in the event of very severe hydroxychloroquine and chloroquine retinopathy.

Fundus Autofluorescence

- Alterations in autofluorescence patterns start early, with a pericentral ring of increased autofluorescence. This ring precedes a mottled loss of autofluorescence in the same area, due to loss of pigment epithelial cells with increased autofluorescence in the adjacent periphery. In more advanced stages, loss of autofluores-

cence at the posterior pole can indicate severe pigment epithelial loss.
- Alterations in autofluorescence precede ophthalmoscopically visible lesions and fluorescein-angiographic abnormalities.

Diagnosis and Treatment

- There has been extensive debate regarding the need for regular screening of patients receiving chloroquine and in particular hydroxychloroquine treatment; recommendations differ between different countries. Recent research has shown that retinal abnormalities are more often found with multifocal electroretinography (mfERG) than previously thought.
- The threat of fast deterioration of visual function, the possible onset of progression after discontinuation of the treatment, and the risk of retinal dysfunction even at low dosage levels in some patients, have to be weighed up against the majority of patients who follow the recommended treatment regimens without developing retinopathy and the impact of regular screening on the health-care system. There is considerable scope for future debate.
- All patients, especially in health-care systems in which regular screening is not recommended, should be informed about early signs of hydroxychloroquine and chloroquine retinopathy.
- MfERG is the most appropriate method for early diagnosis of hydroxychloroquine and chloroquine retinopathy. Initially, pericentral and later generalized amplitude reduction can be observed with mfERG. In small series, mfERG alterations have been reported to precede autofluorescence abnormalities.
- Therapeutically, only the withdrawal of hydroxychloroquine and chloroquine is possible; this should not be carried out abruptly by the ophthalmologist, but in close cooperation with the doctor treating the original disease, in order to avoid exacerbating it.
- Disease progression is possible after withdrawal of hydroxychloroquine and chloroquine; it is unclear whether this is a consequence of the degeneration of the already heavily damaged cells or residual intoxication due to the adsorption of chloroquine into the retinal pigment epithelium.

References

Bienfang D, Coblyn JS, Liang MH, Corzillius M. Hydroxychloroquine retinopathy despite regular ophthalmologic evaluation: a consecutive series. J Rheumatol 2000;27:2703–6.

Kellner U, Kraus H, Foerster MH. Multifocal ERG in chloroquine retinopathy: regional variance of retinal dysfunction. Graefes Arch Clin Exp Ophthalmol 2000;238:94–7.

Marmor MF, Carr RE, Easterbrook M, Farjo AA, Mieler WF. Recommendations on screening for chloroquine and hydroxychloroquine retinopathy. Ophthalmology 2002;109:1377–82.

Maturi RK, Yu M, Weleber RG. Multifocal electroretinographic evaluation of long-term hydroxychloroquine users. Arch Ophthalmol 2004;122: 973–81.

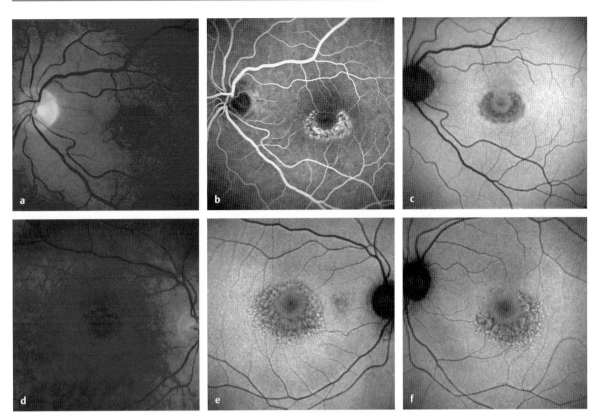

Fig. 4.**7a–f Hydroxychloroquine and chloroquine retinopathy**

a Color photograph. Pericentral pigment epithelial changes in chloroquine retinopathy.

b Arteriovenous phase. Pigment epithelial defects in the area of the clinically visible lesion.

c Fundus autofluorescence. There is reduced autofluorescence in the affected areas.

d Color photograph. Ring-shaped pericentral pigment epithelial changes.

e Fundus autofluorescence. There is a pericentral mottled loss of autofluorescence, consistent with a pigment epithelial defect.

f Fundus autofluorescence (left eye of the same patient as in **d–e**). The changes in this eye are less distinct.

5.1 Choroidal Nevi *Nikolaos E. Bechrakis*

Epidemiology, Pathophysiology, and Clinical Presentation

- Nevi of the choroid are the most common type of intraocular benign tumor, with a prevalence of between 11% and 20%.
- Approximately 90% of choroidal nevi can be found posterior to the equator. They are generally first diagnosed after puberty, once the pigment content has increased.
- The majority of nevi are asymptomatic. Occasionally, however, they can cause functional deficits in the visual field of the overlying retina. In some cases, nevi may show associated serous exudation.
- Drusen often (in approximately 50% of cases) appear on the surface of the nevi, along with chronic degenerative changes in the retinal pigment epithelium, and occasionally (but rarely) choroidal neovascularizations.
- A relatively rare variant of choroidal nevus is melanocytoma, which has very dark to black pigmentation. The most common site of presentation of this type of lesion is on the optic nerve head.

Fluorescein Angiography

- There are no specific angiographic patterns in choroidal nevi. Darkly pigmented nevi generally show a hypofluorescence due to a blockage of the choroidal background fluorescence in all phases of angiography.
- Associated drusen usually show hyperfluorescence. Atrophy of the retinal pigment epithelium appears as a window defect, and accumulations of pigment cause areas of hypofluorescence. Less pigmented or amelanotic nevi may be completely hyperfluorescent. Generally, no visible angiographic microcirculation can be documented in choroidal nevi.

Fundus Autofluorescence

- On fundus autofluorescence, drusen show increased autofluorescence, whereas the other regions of the nevi may either be undetectable by autofluorescence or show spot-like increased autofluorescence. An existing or regressed exudative reaction may be detectable due to increased autofluorescence, typically below the nevi.

Diagnosis and Treatment

- Nevi do not require treatment. The importance of recognizing nevi is the differential diagnosis of small uveal melanocytic lesions.

- Risk factors possibly suggesting growth of a nevus are: tumor width of more than 2.0 mm; juxtapapillary position; symptoms reported by the patient; and the existence of either "orange pigment," subretinal fluid, or complex microcirculation patterns. Fluorescein angiography or indocyanine green angiography are very useful for examining the latter two risk factors and can therefore be informative for assessing or treating small melanocytic lesions.
- Fundus autofluorescence adds further information for differentiating between small choroidal melanoma and nevi. It is always abnormal in choroidal melanoma, often with geographically increased autofluorescence, whereas in choroidal nevi it is often unremarkable or shows more limited alterations.
- Infrared imaging may be helpful for defining the lesion size, which can be difficult to assess with color photography.
- Examination of nevi using optical coherence tomography has revealed a higher incidence of serous exudation (26%) in comparison with ophthalmoscopy. In addition, retinal thinning, retinal edema, retinal pigment epithelial detachment, and photoreceptor attenuation have been noted in association with some nevi.
- Photodynamic therapy has been administered in choroidal neovascularization associated with choroidal nevi, but the results are variable.

References

Parodi MB, Boscia F, Piermarocchi S, et al. Variable outcome of photodynamic therapy for choroidal neovascularization associated with choroidal nevus. Retina 2005;25:438–42.

Shields CL, Cater J, Shields JA, Singh AD, Santos MC, Carvalho C. Combination of clinical factors predictive of growth of small choroidal melanocytic tumors. Arch Ophthalmol 2000;118:360–4.

Shields JA, Mashayekhi A, Ra S, Shields CL. Pseudomelanomas of the posterior uveal tract: the 2006 Taylor R. Smith Lecture. Retina 2005;25:767–71.

Shields CL, Mashayekhi A, Materin MA, et al. Optical coherence tomography of choroidal nevus in 120 patients. Retina 2005;25:243–52.

Singh AD, Kalyani P, Topham A. Estimating the risk of malignant transformation of a choroidal nevus. Ophthalmology 2005;112:1784–9.

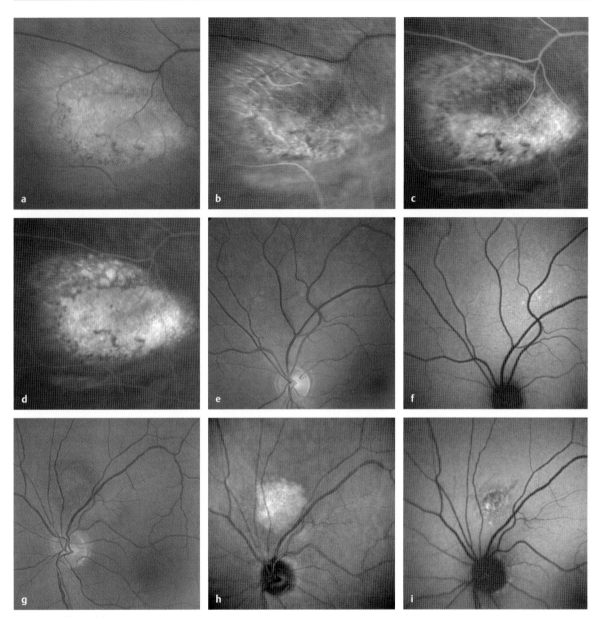

Fig. 5.**1a–i Choroidal nevi**

a Color photograph. Amelanotic choroidal nevus with drusen, discrete atrophies, and accumulation of pigment in the overlying retinal pigment epithelium.

b Early phase. "Normal" choroidal vessels and slight hyperfluorescence of the nevus are visible.

c Arteriovenous phase. There is an increase in the hyperfluorescence, with blockage in the region of the pigment accumulation.

d Late phase. There is a further increase in the hyperfluorescence, including the clinically visible drusen.

e Color photograph. Choroidal nevi near the fovea and superior to the optic disc.

f Fundus autofluorescence. Neither the nevus superior to the optic disc nor the central nevi can be detected. The autofluorescence pattern within the lesions is unremarkable. A few drusen outside are outlined superior to the vascular arcade.

g Color photograph. Small choroidal nevi with a few drusen superior to the optic disc.

h With infrared imaging, the borders of the nevus are more distinct.

i Fundus autofluorescence. In the area of the lesion, spot-like increases in autofluorescence indicate drusen, and some pigment epithelial alterations can be observed.

5.2 Choroidal Melanoma *Nikolaos E. Bechrakis and Lothar Krause*

Epidemiology, Pathophysiology, and Clinical Presentation

- Choroidal melanoma is the most common type of primary malignant intraocular tumor, with an incidence of seven to eight new cases per 1 000 000 in Caucasian populations.
- The 5-year mortality rate averages between 10–50%, depending on the prognostic characteristics of the tumor. Because choroidal melanoma is generally a slow-growing tumor, it is first noticed by the patient when either the tumor directly, or the resultant accompanying exudative detachment, interfere with the fovea or the optic nerve, causing a decrease in visual acuity.
- The more anterior a choroidal melanoma is located, the later the tumor is generally diagnosed.
- Typical diagnostic characteristics of choroidal melanomas are their pigment content, the presence of orange pigment on the surface, an accompanying exudative detachment, and low reflectivity on ultrasonography.

Fluorescein Angiography

- Although choroidal melanomas can have a variety of fluorescein-angiographic characteristics, there are some characteristic patterns that can be indicative of the diagnosis.
- The fluorescein-angiographic image of a choroidal melanoma depends on the size of the tumor, its pigment content, and its interaction with adjacent tissue layers, particularly on the retinal pigment epithelium (RPE) and the retina.
- Generally, early hypofluorescence is seen in pigmented choroidal melanomas, which can change to hyperfluorescence in the later phases of the angiography, depending on the size of the tumor. Flat and less vascularized melanomas can also remain hypofluorescent in the late phase, as long as the RPE has no secondary changes (e. g., through chronic exudation).
- A typical ophthalmoscopic characteristic of choroidal melanomas of any size is the presence of orange pigment on the tumor surface; this consists of lipofuscin accumulation, which, fluorescein angiographically, leads to an earlier, "geographic" blockage of the choroid or tumor hyperfluorescence. In the later phases, these areas can appear hypofluorescent as well as hyperfluorescent; generally, however, the blockage diminishes and produces an image of slowly increasing hyperfluorescence.
- With changes in the RPE, early dot-like areas of hyperfluorescence are typical, which noticeably increase in intensity in the latter phases.
- Occasionally, hemorrhages can be found either on the ophthalmoscopically visible superficial tumor layers between the tumor surface and the intact retina, or epiretinally; depending on length, these lead to different blockages of the underlying fluorescence.

- A typical characteristic in large choroidal melanomas is penetration of the tumors through Bruch membrane, resulting in a mushroom-shaped growth. In these tumors, a characteristic image of "double circulation" can be seen in fluorescein angiography, caused by simultaneously visible retinal and tumor circulations in the early phase, or alternatively in the earlier arteriovenous phase. Hypofluorescence of the larger tumor vessels, with diffuse hyperfluorescence of the surrounding tumor tissue, can be seen during recirculation of the fluorescein in the later phases of the angiography.

Indocyanine Green Angiography

- The anticipated differential-diagnostic relevance of indocyanine green angiography in choroidal tumors has still not been confirmed.
- Early phase. There is hypofluorescence in the melanoma region resulting from the blockage of the choroidal filling through the tumor. Fine vessels can often be seen within the tumor—"double circulation."
- Arteriovenous phase. There is continued blockage of choroidal filling and an appearance of hyperfluorescence in the tumor, as a sign of a leakage from the tumor vessels.
- Late phase. Hyperfluorescence in the tumor increases—a leakage phenomenon.

Fundus Autofluorescence

- Fundus autofluorescence is not useful in large melanomas. In small tumors, which are difficult to differentiate from choroidal nevi, fundus autofluorescence may reveal increased autofluorescence in regions with orange pigment and show flecked alterations in the area of the tumor, in contrast to choroidal nevi. An existing or regressed exudative reaction may be detectable through increased autofluorescence, typically below the small melanoma.

Diagnosis and Treatment

- In general, fluorescein angiography is not of critical importance in the diagnosis of choroidal melanoma and must not be carried out for every intraocular tumor. However, it can provide important information in diagnostically difficult cases, and its contribution is particularly helpful in sparsely pigmented tumors in order to visualize the extent of the tumor and allow treatment planning. It is also helpful for differentiating between nevi and small melanomas (see section 5.1). In addition, it is a useful diagnostic tool for assessing radiation retinopathy (see section 7.11).
- A wide variety of radiotherapy and surgical treatment modalities are available for choroidal melanomas. More detailed articles and textbooks should be consulted for the appropriate treatments.
- Recently, attempts have been made to achieve angiographic imaging of histologically defined and prognos-

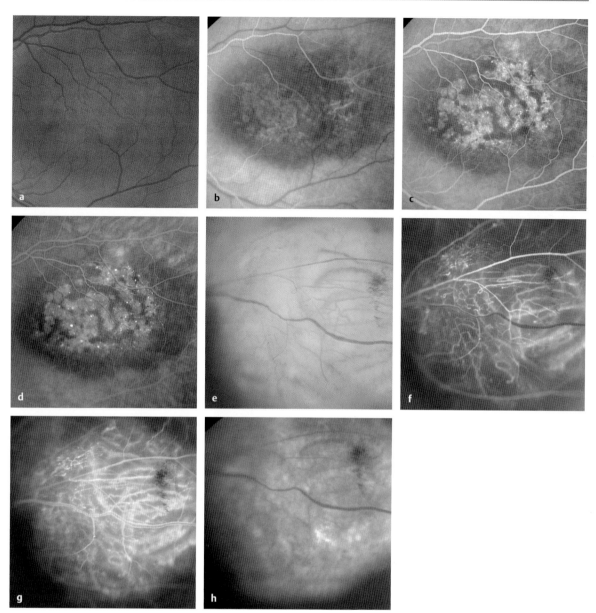

Fig. 5.2a–h   Choroidal melanoma

a Color photograph. A pigmented flat choroidal melanoma with "orange pigment."

b Early phase. Filling of the tumor vessels under the retinal vessels ("double circulation").

c Arteriovenous phase. Hyperfluorescence on the tumor surface, with dot-like "hot spots" and a geographic blockage in the area of the orange pigment.

d Late phase. Further blockage in the area of the orange pigment, and an increase in fluorescence in the hot spots.

e Color photograph. Minimally pigmented large choroidal melanoma with visible large and deep tumor vessels.

f Early phase. Parallel to the arterial filling phase of the retinal vessels, complex microcirculation patterns within the tumor are seen, as well as large tumor vessels.

g Middle phase. Simultaneous depiction of retinal and tumor vessels ("double circulation"). A focal blockage (hypofluorescence) is visible in the region of the tumor surface pigmentation.

h Late phase. An area of diffuse deep hyperfluorescence, as well as several "hot spots," are visible. The large tumor vessels appear hypofluorescent.

tically relevant microcirculation patterns in choroidal melanomas, in order to obtain an additional clinically prognostic parameter. It is not yet clear whether such imaging patterns will have prognostic relevance in everyday practice.

References

Edwards WC, Layden WE, Macdonald R Jr. Fluorescein angiography of malignant melanoma of the choroid. Am J Ophthalmol 1969;68:797–808.

Hayreh SS. Choroidal melanomata: fluorescence angiographic and histopathological study. Br J Ophthalmol 1970;54:145–60.

Krause L, Bechrakis NE, Heinrich S, Kreusel KM, Foerster MH. Indocyanine green angiography and fluorescein angiography of malignant choroidal melanomas following proton beam irradiation. Graefes Arch Clin Exp Ophthalmol 2005:243:545–50.

Mueller AJ, Freeman WR, Schaller UC, Kampik A, Folberg R. Complex microcirculation patterns detected by confocal indocyanine green angiography predict time to growth of small choroidal melanocytic tumors: MuSIC Report II. Ophthalmology 2002;109:2207–14.

Sallet G, Amoaku WM, Lafaut BA, Brabant P, De Laey JJ. Indocyanine green angiography of choroidal tumors. Graefes Arch Clin Exp Ophthalmol 1995;233:677–89.

5

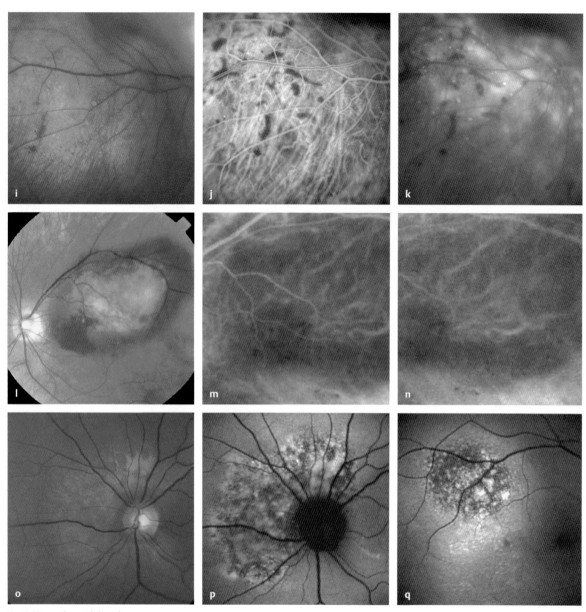

Fig. 5.**2i–q Choroidal melanoma**

i Color photograph. A moderately pigmented large choroidal melanoma, with orange pigment on the surface.

j Middle phase. Geographic blockages in areas with orange pigment and dot-like hot spots.

k Late phase. The deep diffuse focal hyperfluorescence in the tumor makes the retinal and tumor vessels appear hypofluorescent.

l Color photograph. Malignant melanoma of the choroid, with orange pigment on the tumor surface. The tumor has variably strong pigmentation.

m Indocyanine green angiography, early phase. The blockage of choroidal filling by the tumor is clearly recognizable. The retinal vessels are already filled. A vascular network can be seen within the tumor, which cannot be assigned either to the choroidal vessels or the retinal vessels.

n Indocyanine green angiography, late phase. In contrast to fluorescein angiography, there is virtually no leakage within the tumor. The tumor vessels are therefore still easily recognized. In addition, the tumor is continuing to block choroidal filling.

o Color photograph. A small juxtapapillary choroidal melanoma with orange pigment.

p Fundus autofluorescence. Increased autofluorescence in regions with orange pigment and flecked retinal pigment epithelial alterations in the area of the tumor.

q Fundus autofluorescence (in a different patient). There is increased autofluorescence, corresponding to orange pigment, flecked retinal pigment epithelial alterations, and increased autofluorescence below the small melanoma due to an exudative reaction.

5.3 Choroidal Hemangioma
Klaus-Martin Kreusel and Lothar Krause

Epidemiology, Pathophysiology, and Clinical Presentation

- Localized choroidal hemangiomas should be differentiated from diffuse choroidal hemangiomas.
- Diffuse choroidal hemangiomas appear in conjunction with Sturge–Weber syndrome. They can partially or completely affect the choroid; the choroid is diffusely thicker in the tumor region and has a deep red color ("ketchup" fundus). Ipsilaterally, a secondary glaucoma is often present, as well as nevus flammeus on the facial skin and also a leptomeningeal hemangioma. Diffuse choroidal hemangiomas often already become symptomatic in childhood with an exudative retinal detachment.
- Localized choroidal hemangiomas appear in otherwise healthy patients, become symptomatic in middle age, are almost always solitary, and are located central to the equator. They appear as prominent, raspberry-colored subretinal tumors. In addition, there may also be secondary pigment alterations, macular edema, and exudative retinal detachment.
- Both types of choroidal hemangioma are subtypes of hamartomas and do not usually show any increase in size. Histologically, they consist of cavernous and capillary vascular networks.

Fluorescein Angiography

- Localized choroidal hemangiomas have a characteristic fluorescein-angiographic image that is indicative of the diagnosis.
- Very rapid filling of the angioma takes place after injection of fluorescein, and the tumor's vessel system can be identified before filling of the retinal vessels. Fundus photography has to be started immediately after fluorescein injection in order to establish the early filling of the hemangioma that is essential for the diagnosis.
- In the course of the angiography, a clear depiction of the hemangioma vessel system is initially seen, followed by increasing dye leakage from the hemangioma, causing an increasing diffuse hyperfluorescence in the tumor area.
- Fluorescein angiography is of no value in the diagnosis of diffuse choroidal hemangiomas.

Indocyanine Green Angiography

- The anticipated differential-diagnostic relevance of indocyanine green angiography in choroidal tumors has still not been confirmed.

- Early phase. Typically, there is very early hyperfluorescence in the hemangioma area due to large intratumoral vessels.
- Arteriovenous phase. There is increasing hyperfluorescence in the tumor area.
- Late phase. There is hyperfluorescence in the tumor increases, and dye appears in the choroidal vessels and causes a diffuse hyperfluorescence in the tumor.

Diagnosis and Treatment

- Localized choroidal hemangiomas can sometimes be difficult to detect with ophthalmoscopy, but they are usually recognizable in stereoscopic images due to their prominence. Secondary pigment epithelium changes can complicate the diagnostic differentiation of choroidal melanoma.
- Fluorescein angiography is essential for diagnosing and determining the extent of localized choroidal hemangiomas.
- Characteristic ophthalmoscopy images, together with the additional organ lesions that are almost always detectable in patients with Sturge–Weber syndrome, are the key characteristics required for the diagnosis of diffuse choroidal hemangioma.
- Additional diagnostic measures include ultrasonography and high-resolution magnetic resonance imaging of the orbit, which can be useful in the differential diagnosis of choroidal melanoma.
- Therapeutically, external radiotherapy using photons or protons, laser therapy using argon or diode laser, and photodynamic therapy can be administered. Recent reports suggest that photodynamic therapy is the treatment of choice in localized choroidal hemangioma.

References

Anand R, Augsburger JJ, Shields JA. Circumscribed choroidal hemangiomas. Arch Ophthalmol 1989;107:1338–42.

Jurklies B, Bornfeld N. The role of photodynamic therapy in the treatment of symptomatic choroidal hemangioma. Graefe Arch Clin Exp Ophthalmol 2005;243:393–6.

Schilling H, Sauerwein W, Lommatzsch A, et al. Long-term results after low dose ocular irradiation for choroidal haemangiomas. Br J Ophthalmol 1997;81:267–73.

Stroszczynski C, Hosten N, Bornfeld N, et al. Choroidal hemangioma: MR findings and differentiation from uveal melanoma. AJNR Am J Neuroradiol 1998;19:1441–7.

Sullivan TJ, Clarke MP, Morin JD. The ocular manifestations of the Sturge–Weber syndrome. J Pediatr Ophthalmol Strabismus 1992;29:349–56.

Wessing A. Fluorescein-angiography and the differential diagnosis of choroidal tumors. Bull Soc Belge Ophtalmol 1977;175:5–14.

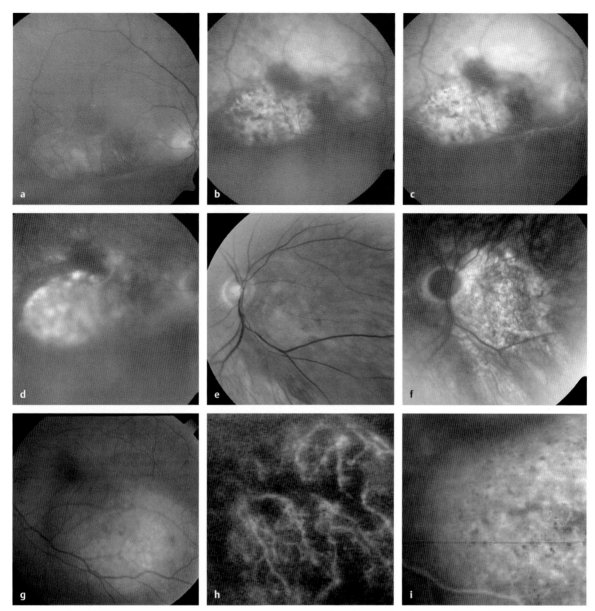

5

Fig. 5.**3a–i Choroidal hemangioma**

a Color photograph. Circumscribed choroidal hemangioma in the macula, extending from below up to the fovea, with an accompanying exudative retinal detachment extending to the optic nerve head. In comparison with normal tissue, the somewhat darker coloring of this hemangioma makes it ophthalmoscopically visible.

b Early phase. The hemangioma's vascular system—a large, mesh-like vascular pattern with variations in caliber—is already visible before filling of the retinal vessel system.

c Early phase. The retinal vessels are starting to fill. An increasing nonuniform hyperfluorescence in the tumor region is visible due to the accumulation of the fluorescein in the cavernous regions of the hemangioma, as well as leakage from the hemangioma vessels.

d Late phase. There is a further increase in spotty hyperfluorescence in the tumor region, reflecting the intravascular and extravascular accumulation of fluorescein.

e Color photograph. There is a localized juxtapapillary hemangioma nasal to the optic nerve head, which is ophthalmoscopically identifiable due to its slightly lighter and spotty fundus appearance and its prominence in the stereoscopic image.

f Late phase. The persistent hyperfluorescence corresponds to the surface extension of the hemangioma.

g Color photograph. A choroidal hemangioma in a typical location at the posterior pole of the eye. Ophthalmoscopically, this tumor appears red.

h Indocyanine green angiography, early phase. The very early filling of the tumor is characteristic of choroidal hemangioma. In the earlier phase, the choroidal filling suggests there is no blockage. The vessels within the tumor are clearly recognizable.

i Indocyanine green angiography, late phase. There is an increase in hyperfluorescence in the tumor, reflecting increasing leakage. The hemangioma continues to be hyperfluorescent, while fluorescence decreases in the rest of the choroid.

5.4 Retinal Capillary Angioma
Klaus-Martin Kreusel

Epidemiology, Pathophysiology, and Clinical Presentation

- Retinal capillary angiomas are slow-growing, benign retinal tumors that arise from proliferated capillaries and neuroglia. They are mainly associated with von Hippel–Lindau syndrome, an autosomal-dominant multitumor syndrome with a prevalence of one in 40 000, and, in the majority of cases, are multiple and bilateral. More rarely, nonsyndromic (but always solitary) angiomas can be observed.
- Large peripheral angiomas have a typical ophthalmoscopic appearance, with conspicuously dilated and tortuous afferent vessels ("feeder vessels").
- Juxtapapillary angiomas have a less typical picture. The endophytic, intraretinal, or exophytic appearances can vary.
- In large and/or multiple tumors, secondary changes such as macular edema, epiretinal membranes, tractional, and/or exudative retinal detachments are the symptoms leading to clinical presentation.

Fluorescein Angiography

- In peripheral angiomas, conspicuously extended afferent and efferent vessels can be seen, correlating with the size of the angioma. Due to the higher blood flow, these vessels can fill more quickly than the surrounding normal retinal vessels in the early phase.
- In larger angiomas, an early hyperfluorescence in the region of the angioma, which increases throughout the later phases, can be seen. The feeder vessels do not usually show any signs of fluorescein leakage.
- It is generally not possible to differentiate the capillary structure of peripheral angiomas angiographically, but it can sometimes be seen in a juxtapapillary angioma.
- The surrounding retinal vessel system is usually unremarkable.
- Juxtapapillary angiomas usually fill at the same time as, or even after, the filling of the arterial retinal vessels. This is an important angiographic criterion for the diagnostic differentiation of juxtapapillary choroid hemangiomas (which usually fill simultaneously with the choroid vessels, before the retinal circulation).

Diagnosis and Treatment

- The diagnosis of peripheral angiomas can generally be established on the basis of their typical ophthalmoscopic appearance. Fluorescein angiography can be helpful in the diagnosis and documentation of small angiomas and makes a decisive contribution to the differential diagnostic classification of juxtapapillary angiomas.
- The patient's history and family history should be carefully investigated for any cases of von Hippel–Lindau syndrome; genetic counseling and assessment for the *VHL* gene are advisable. If there is any suspicion or evidence of von Hippel–Lindau syndrome, extensive and regular check-ups are indicated to allow early detection of additional organ manifestations (e. g., hemangioblastoma of the central nervous system, abdominal tumors).
- Therapy depends on the size and location of the angioma and the associated secondary changes; argon laser coagulation, transpupillary thermotherapy, brachytherapy, or vitrectomy can all be considered as treatment measures. Therapy for juxtapapillary angiomas is more difficult; in these cases, proton-beam therapy or photodynamic therapy can be considered.

References

Gass JD, Braunstein R. Sessile and exophytic capillary angiomas of the juxtapapillary retina and optic nerve head. Arch Ophthalmol 1980;98:1790–7.

Grossniklaus HE, Thomas JW, Vigneswaran N, Jarrett WH 3rd. Retinal hemangioblastoma: a histologic, immunohistochemical, and ultrastructural evaluation. Ophthalmology 1992;99:140–5.

Kreusel KM, Bornfeld N, Lommatzsch A, Wessing A, Foerster MH. Ruthenium-106 brachytherapy for peripheral retinal capillary hemangioma. Ophthalmology 1998;105:1386–92.

Kreusel KM, Bechrakis NE, Heinichen T, Neumann L, Neumann HP, Foerster MH. Retinal angiomatosis and von Hippel–Lindau disease. Graefes Arch Clin Exp Ophthalmol 2000;238:916–21.

Neumann HP, Lips CJ, Hsia YE, Zbar B. Von Hippel–Lindau syndrome. Brain Pathol 1995;5:181–93.

5

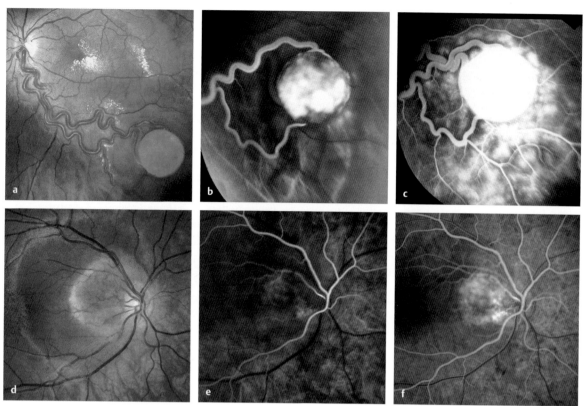

Fig. 5.4a–f Retinal capillary angioma

a Color photograph. A large peripheral angioma with massively dilated afferent and efferent retinal vessels. Characteristic lipid exudates can be seen in the macula, at some distance from the tumor.

b Early phase. There is rapid but irregular filling of the angioma through the afferent arteries.

c Arteriovenous phase. The start of fluorescein leakage from the angioma, which can increase considerably in the later phases of angiography.

d Color photograph. A juxtapapillary intraretinal angioma on the temporal edge of the optic nerve head, with detachment of the neurosensory retina in the macula.

e Early phase. Filling of the angioma takes place after filling of the retinal arteries. The capillary structure of the tumor can be identified.

f Early arteriovenous phase. The angioma is completely filled with fluorescein, in the later phases; increasing leakage of dye into the macula can be seen.

5

5.5 Astrocytoma   *Klaus-Martin Kreusel*

Epidemiology, Pathophysiology, and Clinical Presentation

- Astrocytomas are retinal hamartomas that often appear in the context of tuberous sclerosis (Bourneville–Pringle disease), occasionally sporadically or in type 1 neurofibromatosis.
- Astrocytomas are rarely progressive and are almost always asymptomatic. They are located in the inner retinal layers, typically obscuring the retinal vessels. They may present as solitary or multiple lesions, in juxtapapillary locations or on the periphery of the retina. A fluffy appearance is more common than the typical mulberry aspect, which indicates the cystic degeneration of the tumor. Transformation from the fluffy to mulberry type can also take place.
- Histologically, astrocytomas consist of spindle-shaped or pleomorphic astrocytes with a vascular network. Various grades of calcification, as well as cystoid cavities, can also exist.
- Retinal astrocytoma is present in approximately 50% of patients with tuberous sclerosis. Other signs of this autosomal-dominant syndrome (with a prevalence of one in 10 000), which becomes symptomatic in childhood, are skin lesions (plaque, hypopigmentation), central nervous system changes (tuber, calcification) that can lead to retardation and epilepsy, and visceral tumors (cardiac rhabdomyoma, renal angiomyolipoma, renal cysts).
- Molecular-genetic analysis has shown associated mutations in two genes (*TSC1* and *TSC2*), the gene products of which play an important part in several cell-signaling pathways.

Fluorescein Angiography

- In the early phase, there is blockage of the background fluorescence by the tumor mass. The retinal vessels may be partly translucent.
- In the middle phase, a delicate basal vascular network may be seen inside the tumor, but this is not always clearly visible due to the overlying avascular tumor tissue. The vessel density in the fluffy type is higher than that in the mulberry type.
- In the late phase, leakage from the tumor vessels takes place, leading to increasing hyperfluorescence of the tumor and veiling of the tumor's vascular network.

Diagnosis and Treatment

- Mulberry-type astrocytomas are easy to recognize owing to their typical ophthalmoscopic features.
- Fluffy-type astrocytomas have to be differentiated ophthalmoscopically from retinoblastomas. There are no clear fluorescein-angiographic criteria for distinguishing between the two entities.
- Additional organ manifestations of tuberous sclerosis, such as neonatal convulsions or skin manifestation ("white spots"), as well as a positive family history, can be important for differentiating the condition from retinoblastoma. Pathognomonic adenoma sebaceum first appears in puberty.
- In contrast to retinoblastoma, astrocytomas are almost always inactive. This means that vitreous infiltration, retinal detachment, hemorrhage, and retinal necrosis are rare. However, vitreous hemorrhage has been reported in a number of individual cases.
- Treatment for astrocytoma is not necessary. Pediatric and neurological examinations, as well as genetic counseling, are advisable if the presence of tuberous sclerosis is suspected.

References

Roach ES, Sparagana SP. Diagnosis of tuberous sclerosis complex. J Child Neurol 2004;19:643–9.

Shields JA, Eagle RC Jr, Shields CL, Marr BP. Aggressive retinal astrocytoma in four patients with tuberous sclerosis complex. Trans Am Ophthalmol Soc 2004;102:139–47.

Zimmer-Galler IE, Robertson DM. Long-term observation of retinal lesions in tuberous sclerosis. Am J Ophthalmol 1995;119:318–24.

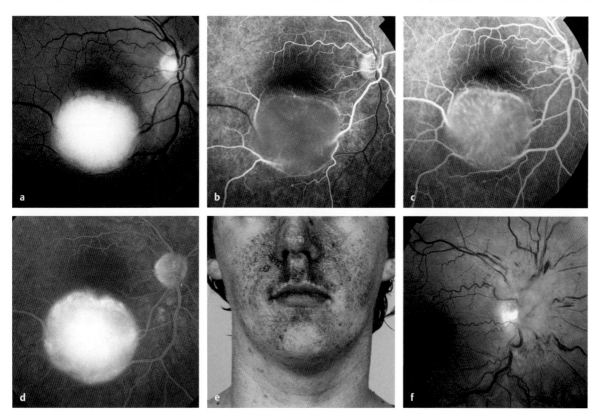

Fig. 5.**5a–f Astrocytoma**

a Color photograph. Sporadic astrocytoma in the temporal lower vessel arcade, with a suggestion of a mulberry-type structure at the central edge of the tumor. This tumor is located in the inner retinal layers; the retinal vessels are obscured.

b Early arteriovenous phase. There is relative blockage of the background fluorescence in the tumor region, on the edge of which translucent retinal vessels can be seen.

c Late arteriovenous phase. There is a distinct vascular system within the tumor. The vessels appear diffuse, as they are located in the basal part of the tumor and the overlying tumor mass is obscuring them.

d Late phase. There is persistent hyperfluorescence in the tumor area due to fluorescein leakage from the tumor vessels.

e Adenoma sebaceum of the facial skin in tuberous sclerosis. This pathognomonic stigma first appears in puberty.

f Juxtapapillary astrocytoma of the fluffy type (in same patient as in **e**). This type of astrocytoma has a less characteristic appearance than the mulberry variety.

5

5.6 Choroidal Metastasis   *Klaus-Martin Kreusel and Lothar Krause*

Epidemiology, Pathophysiology, and Clinical Presentation

- The choroid is by far the most common location for intraocular metastases. Choroidal metastases appear in approximately 10% of advanced cases of carcinomatous diseases and are thus the most common intraocular tumor. However, symptomatic choroidal metastases are much more rare than primary choroidal melanoma.
- Clinically, the most common primary tumor is previously diagnosed breast cancer. However, choroidal metastases can occasionally be the first clinical sign of the malignant disease; in most of these cases, a bronchial carcinoma can subsequently be diagnosed.
- Funduscopically, choroidal metastasis typically present as multiple, flat, pale, or cream-colored lesions central to the equator.
- Rarely, choroidal metastases appear as highly prominent pigmented tumors with accompanying retinal detachment. The differential diagnosis from primary choroidal melanoma can sometimes be difficult in these cases.

Fluorescein Angiography

- Choroidal metastases do not have specific, characteristic angiographic patterns.
- Flat lesions show blockage of the background fluorescence in the early phases of angiography; mild hyperfluorescence is possible in the late phase.
- In thicker lesions, the tumor may have its own vascular network, and stronger leakage of the dye is also visible.

Indocyanine Green Angiography

- The anticipated differential-diagnostic relevance of indocyanine green angiography in choroidal tumors has not yet been confirmed.
- Early phase. There is hypofluorescence in the metastasis area, due to blockage of choroidal filling by the tumor. In the majority of cases, no vessels can be seen within the tumor.

- Arteriovenous phase. There is continued blockage of choroid filling. Hyperfluorescence appears in the tumor as an expression of pigment epithelial defects.
- Late phase. The hyperfluorescence in the tumor increases.

Diagnosis and Treatment

- In patients with previously diagnosed metastatic cancer and typical multiple choroidal lesions, it is possible to base the diagnosis on ophthalmoscopy alone.
- In solitary, highly prominent metastases, definite differentiation from choroidal melanoma is not possible using ophthalmoscopy.
- The diagnosis is usually confirmed by verifying the primary tumor, or possibly on the basis of other organ metastases in patients with previously identified tumor disease. Intraocular biopsy may be appropriate in situations in which the diagnosis cannot be established with conventional methods.
- The standard therapy is teletherapy, with external beam radiotherapy; brachytherapy with a radioactive plaque can also be used in large solitary metastases.

References

Albert DM, Rubenstein RA, Scheie HG. Tumor metastasis to the eye, 1: incidence in 213 adult patients with generalized malignancy. Am J Ophthalmol 1967;63:723–6.

Bechrakis NE, Foerster MH, Bornfeld N. Biopsy in indeterminate intraocular tumors. Ophthalmology 2002;109:235–42.

Krause L, Bechrakis NE, Kreusel KM, Servetopoulou F, Heinrich S, Foerster MH. Indocyanine green angiography in choroid metastases; in German. Ophthalmologe 2002;99:617–9.

Kreusel KM, Wiegel T, Stange M, et al. Choroidal metastasis in disseminated lung cancer: frequency and risk factors. Am J Ophthalmol 2002;134:445–7.

Shields CL, Shields JA, Gross NE, Schwartz GP, Lally SE. Survey of 520 eyes with uveal metastases. Ophthalmology 1997;104:1265–76.

Wiegel T, Bottke D, Kreusel KM, et al. External beam radiotherapy of choroidal metastases: final results of a prospective study of the German Cancer Society (ARO 95–08). Radiother Oncol 2002;64:13–8.

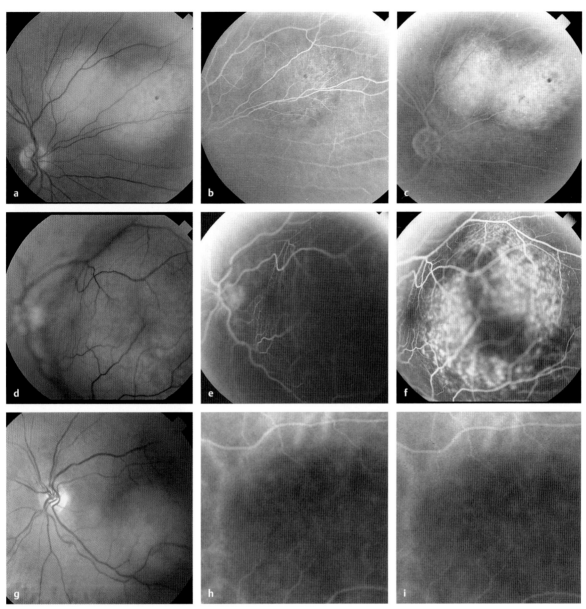

Fig. 5.**6a–i Choroidal metastasis**

a Color photograph. Confluent flat, amelanotic choroidal metastasis associated with an adenocarcinoma of unknown origin.

b Arteriovenous phase. Discrete spotty hyperfluorescence in the tumor area; no evidence of a tumor vessel system.

c Late phase. Persisting hyperfluorescence without significant dye leakage in the tumor area.

d Color photograph. Highly prominent choroidal metastasis at the posterior pole from a bronchial carcinoma reaching from temporal up to the fovea.

e Early arteriovenous phase. Complete blockage of the background fluorescence in the tumor area, the tumor's own vessel system is still not identifiable.

f Late arteriovenous phase. A tumor with its own vessel system with aneurysmatic expanded capillaries can be seen; followed later by increasing dye leakage from the vessels.

g Color photograph. The picture shows a choroidal metastasis at the temporal lower vessel arcade. An accumulation of pigment is often visible ophthalmoscopically, so that the tumors have a speckled appearance. An accompanying retinal detachment mostly occurs in larger metastases.

h Indocyanine green (ICG) angiography, middle phase. Blockage of the choroidal filling by the metastasis, intra-tumoral vessels do not occur. Fine-flecked hyperfluorescences can be seen within the metastasis.

i ICG angiography, late phase. In the late phase, clear blockage of the choroidal filling takes place. The flecked shaped hyperfluorescences increase somewhat in intensity, clear leakages cannot be seen.

5.7 Vasoproliferative Tumors   *Klaus-Martin Kreusel*

Epidemiology, Pathophysiology, and Clinical Presentation

- Vasoproliferative tumors are rare, benign retinal tumors of unclear etiology. They mainly appear as unilateral and solitary lesions, but multiple lesions may also occur.
- Otherwise healthy patients aged between 40 and 60 years are mainly affected, possibly with a genetic predisposition.
- In approximately one-quarter of cases, there is an association with another ocular disease, such as uveitis, retinitis pigmentosa, retinopathy of prematurity, retinochoroiditis, sickle-cell retinopathy, or a long-standing retinal detachment.
- Vasoproliferative tumors are mainly found in the lower periphery in the form of prominent, yellow to red lesions with only slightly dilated, occasionally multiple afferent and efferent vessels. They often have distinct lipid exudates around the tumor (which can even have the appearance of pseudotumors), marked reactive pigment epithelial changes, as well as retinal hemorrhages, and occasionally also vitreous hemorrhages.
- The tumors often become symptomatic either due to secondary macular edema or vitreous hemorrhage, or, in advanced stages, due to exudative or tractional retinal detachment.
- Histologically, proliferative neuroglia cells, in association with a capillary vascular network that is sometimes telangiectatic, can be found.

Fluorescein Angiography

- Angiography makes it possible to confirm the vascular nature of the tumor. The afferent arteries can be visualized in the early phase. It is also often possible to distinguish the capillary intratumoral vascular system.
- In the later phases, the efferent veins can be seen, along with increasing diffuse leakage from the tumor vessels.
- Angiographically, the tumor structure often appears inhomogeneous, with looser and denser capillary structures in some areas.
- In the majority of cases, an intratumoral dilation of telangiectatic vessels is visible.

Diagnosis and Treatment

- The diagnosis is based on the ophthalmoscopic and angiographic features.
- The differential diagnosis from capillary retinal angioma can be difficult. Capillary retinal angiomas occur in patients who are on average younger, and mainly in the context of von Hippel–Lindau syndrome; the lesions generally have dilated, tortuous afferent and efferent vessels and a well-defined hemispherical tumor structure.
- Von Hippel–Lindau syndrome should be excluded through the clinical examination or family history, if possible; otherwise, molecular-genetic examinations should be considered (see section 5.4).
- The treatment of vasoproliferative tumors is based on the size of the lesion and the existence of secondary complications.
- In small lesions, argon laser coagulation or transpupillary thermotherapy can be used; in peripherally located tumors, cryotherapy can also be employed. Brachytherapy or cryotherapy should be considered in patients with larger lesions.
- Vitrectomy can be considered when there are secondary changes, such as traction membranes, macular pucker, or marked exudative retinal detachment.

References

Heimann H, Bornfeld N, Vij O, et al. Vasoproliferative tumours of the retina. Br J Ophthalmol 2000;84:1162–9.

Irvine F, O'Donnell N, Kemp E, Lee WR. Retinal vasoproliferative tumors: surgical management and histological findings. Arch Ophthalmol 2000;118:563–9.

Shields CL, Shields JA, Barrett J, De Potter P. Vasoproliferative tumors of the ocular fundus: classification and clinical manifestations in 103 patients. Arch Ophthalmol 1995;113:615–23.

Wachtlin J, Heimann H, Jandeck C, et al. Bilateral vasoproliferative retinal tumors with identical localization in a pair of monozygotic twins. Arch Ophthalmol 2002;120:860–2.

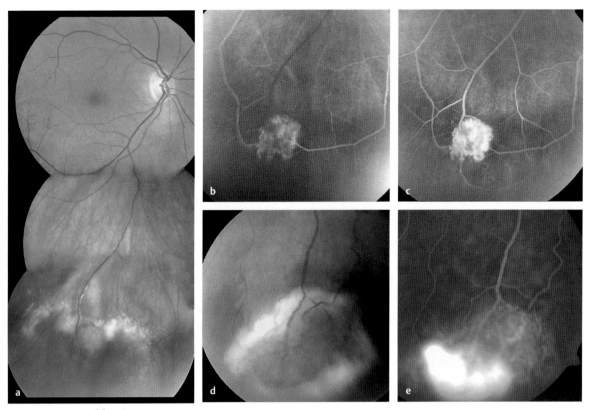

Fig. 5.**7a–e Vasoproliferative tumors**

a Color photograph. There is a vasoproliferative tumor in the lower periphery, with only minimally dilated afferent vessels and with surrounding lipid exudates.

b Early phase. Two afferent arterial vessels can be seen on each side of the tumor; the capillary structure of the tumor is easily recognized.

c Late arteriovenous phase. Increasing dye leakage from the tumor is developing, making the details and borders of the tumor increasingly difficult to distinguish.

d Color photograph. There is a large fibrovascular tumor in the lower periphery, with lipid exudates surrounding it. The afferent artery has a tortuous appearance, and the efferent vein shows increased filling and caliber fluctuations.

e Late phase of **d**. The angiogram shows the inhomogeneous internal structure of the tumor clearly. There is a more solid part with no distinguishable vascular structures and clear dye leakage, and another part that has a clearly recognizable dilated capillary network with telangiectasis.

6.1 Nonproliferative Diabetic Retinopathy   *Horst Helbig*

Epidemiology, Pathophysiology, and Clinical Presentation

- Diabetic retinopathy occurs in 98% of patients with type 1 diabetes after 15 years of diabetes, in approximately 55% of those with type 2 diabetes not receiving insulin treatment, and in approximately 85% of those with type 2 diabetes receiving insulin treatment.
- The basic pathophysiological alterations relate to increased permeability as well as occlusion of the retinal capillaries, leading to the development of retinal edema and reduced perfusion and ischemia of the retina, resulting in deterioration of retinal function.
- Nonproliferative diabetic retinopathy (NPDR) is classified according to its severity:
  - Mild NPDR: microaneurysms
  - Moderate NPDR: additional retinal hemorrhage, cotton-wool spots
  - Severe NPDR: additional larger hemorrhages in four quadrants, venous beading in two quadrants, or distinct intraretinal microvascular anomalies (IRMAs)

Fluorescein Angiography

- Microaneurysms appear as dot-like areas of hyperfluorescence, or may appear hypofluorescent if they have thrombosed.
- Retinal hemorrhages and hard exudates block the choroid fluorescence.
- In the majority of cases, capillary occlusions can only be identified angiographically. Vessels adjacent to nonperfused areas often show increased permeability.
- Increased permeability of retinal capillaries is angiographically characterized as ill-defined hyperfluorescence in the vessel wall. In late images, the adjacent edematous retinal tissue is diffusely stained.
- Cotton-wool spots represent swollen nerve fibers in the area of micro-infarctions of the inner retina, and have a hypofluorescent appearance due to blockage of the choroidal fluorescence by the opaque nerve fibers and due to the underlying retinal capillary occlusion.
- Intraretinal microvascular abnormalities are dilated and tortuous preexisting capillaries, or may be newly formed intraretinal vessels. As with localized areas of venous beading, they typically occur next to areas of capillary occlusion.

Diagnosis and Treatment

- The diagnosis is established by clinical examination with binocular ophthalmoscopy. Angiography is not obligatory.
- Optimization of blood pressure and the blood glucose level delays the development of diabetic retinopathy and progression to proliferative retinopathy in both type 1 and type 2 diabetes.
- Mild scatter laser coagulation can be considered in severe nonproliferative diabetic retinopathy (NPDR), particularly when there is proliferative retinopathy in the fellow eye or if poor compliance with check-up examinations is expected.

References

Bornfeld N, Joussen AM, Helbig H, et al. Augenerkrankungen. In: Mehnert H, Standl E, Usadel KH, editors. Diabetologie in Klinik und Praxis, 5th ed. Stuttgart: Thieme, 2003: 523–49.

Cunha-Vaz J, Bernardes R. Nonproliferative retinopathy in diabetes type 2: initial stages and characterization of phenotypes. Prog Retin Eye Res 2005;24:355–77.

Flynn HW, Smiddy WE. Diabetes and ocular disease: past, present, and future therapies. San Francisco: Foundation of the American Academy of Ophthalmology, 2000 (Ophthalmology Monographs, 14).

Hamilton AMP, Ulbig MW, Polkinghorne P. Management of diabetic retinopathy. London: British Medical Journal Publishing Group, 1996.

Wilkinson CP, Ferris FL 3rd, Klein RE, et al. Proposed international clinical diabetic retinopathy and diabetic macular edema disease severity scales. Ophthalmology 2003;110:1677–82.

6

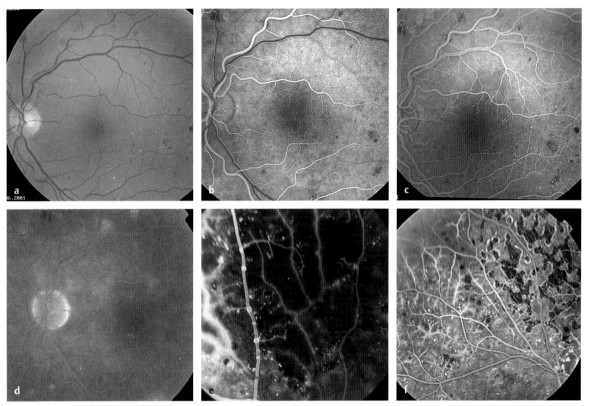

Fig. 6.**1a–f Nonproliferative diabetic retinopathy**

a Color photograph. Moderate nonproliferative diabetic retinopathy with small retinal hemorrhages, microaneurysms, and hard exudates.

b Early arteriovenous phase. Blockage of the background fluorescence caused by retinal hemorrhages.

c Arteriovenous phase. Dot-like hyperfluorescence of the microaneurysms.

d Late phase. Areas of mild hyperfluorescence in a region with permeable capillaries and microaneurysms, reflecting localized retinal edema.

e Arteriovenous phase (in a different patient). Severe nonproliferative diabetic retinopathy with extensive areas of capillary occlusion and venous beading.

f Arteriovenous phase (in a different patient). The effect of laser coagulation on an ischemic retina. Retinal areas with capillary occlusion and ill-defined staining of the vessels, reflecting increased vessel wall permeability, can be seen on the left of the image. An area with laser scars can be seen on the right; in this area, only the vessel lumina stain, with no dye leakage.

6

6.2 Diabetic Macular Edema   *Horst Helbig*

Epidemiology, Pathophysiology, and Clinical Presentation

- Macular edema is responsible for the majority of visual loss in diabetic retinopathy, particularly in patients with type 2 diabetes. Functional loss develops as a result of swelling of the central retina.
- Diabetic macular edemas are clinically divided into the following subgroups:
  - Focal diabetic macular edema
  - Diffuse diabetic macular edema
  - Ischemic diabetic maculopathy
  - Mixed forms

Fluorescein Angiography

- Macular edema occurs as a result of leakage of fluid from hyperpermeable capillary walls into the adjacent macular tissue. These capillaries are also permeable to fluorescein, which during angiography initially stains the vessel walls and then in the late phase stains the swollen retinal tissue.
- The perifoveal capillary arcades show rarefaction and ectatic changes in the retinal capillaries, as a sign of incipient central ischemia. Laser coagulation is not advisable in cases of marked central ischemia. Angiography is recommended before laser coagulation of diffuse macular edema.
- Angiographically, diffuse macular edema often shows cystoid components.

Diagnosis and Treatment

- The indication for central laser coagulation is based on the presence of what is known as "clinically significant macular edema." According to the Early Treatment Diabetic Retinopathy Study Research Group (ETDRS), macular edema can be described as clinically significant if the swelling of the retina and hard exudates is less than 500 μm from the center of the fovea, or if the region of swelling is larger than one disk diameter and is less than one disk diameter away from the center. The diagnosis is established by clinical stereoscopic ophthalmoscopy of the macula (not by fluorescein angiography).
- Laser treatment rarely leads to improvement in visual acuity. The aim of laser treatment is to achieve stabilization or to delay deterioration. If macular edema and proliferative retinopathy present simultaneously, the macular edema should be treated first.
- In focal macular edema, the circumscribed area of swollen retina should be coagulated in a targeted way, including the leaking microaneurysms and the capillaries.
- In diffuse macular edema, the macula around the fovea should be coagulated in a grid-like fashion.
- Laser treatment is not beneficial for advanced ischemic maculopathy. However, ischemic zones in the peripheral macula should be coagulated.
- Any supplementary central laser coagulation that may be needed after the initial treatment should not be carried out before 3 months have elapsed. At check-up examinations, the hard exudates may have "condensed" and thus appear to have increased. Reabsorption of hard exudates during or after regression of the edema may take months or years.
- Therapeutic approaches currently under investigation include intravitreal application of various drugs—e. g., corticosteroids and antiangiogenic agents—and macular surgery (vitrectomy with removal of the internal limiting membrane). Intravitreal injection of triamcinolone acetonide and other drugs have replaced grid laser for the treatment of diffuse diabetic macular edema in many retinal centers.
- Optical coherence tomography (OCT, Zeiss, Germany), a Retinal Thickness Analyzer (RTA, Talia, Israel), or the macular module of the Heidelberg Retina Tomograph (HRT, Heidelberg Engineering, Germany) can be used to measure retinal thickness in diabetic macular edema before and after treatment. Although the different methods may be difficult to compare, reliable follow-up measurements are possible with the same method and are less invasive than repeated fluorescein angiographies.
- Early detection of subclinical diabetic macular edema is facilitated by OCT imaging.

References

Avitabile T, Longo A, Reibaldi A. Intravitreal triamcinolone compared with macular laser grid photocoagulation for the treatment of cystoid macular edema. Am J Ophthalmol 2005;140:695–702

Browning DJ, McOwen MD, Bowen RM Jr, O'Marah TL. Comparison of the clinical diagnosis of diabetic macular edema with diagnosis by optical coherence tomography. Ophthalmology 2004;111:712–5.

Chew EY, Ferris FL 3rd, Csaky KG, et al. The long-term effects of laser photocoagulation treatment in patients with diabetic retinopathy: the early treatment diabetic retinopathy follow-up study. Ophthalmology 2003;110:1683–9.

Cunningham ET Jr, Adamis AP, Altaweel M, et al: A phase II randomized double-masked trial of pegaptanib, an anti-vascular endothelial growth factor aptamer, for diabetic macular edema. Ophthalmology 2005;112:1747–57

Early Treatment Diabetic Retinopathy Study Research Group. Early photocoagulation for diabetic retinopathy. ETDRS report number 9. Ophthalmology 1991;98:766–85.

Early Treatment Diabetic Retinopathy Study Research Group. Focal photocoagulation treatment of diabetic macular edema: relationship of treatment effect to fluorescein angiographic and other retinal characteristics at baseline. ETDRS report no. 19. Arch Ophthalmol 1995;113:1144–55.

Sutter FK, Simpson JM, Gillies MC. Intravitreal triamcinolone for diabetic macular edema that persists after laser treatment: three-month efficacy and safety results of a prospective, randomized, double-masked, placebo-controlled clinical trial. Ophthalmology 2004;111:2044–9.

Tranos PG, Wickremasinghe SS, Stangos NT, et al. Macular edema. Surv Ophthalmol 2004;49:470–90.

Wilkinson CP, Ferris FL 3rd, Klein RE, et al. Proposed international clinical diabetic retinopathy and diabetic macular edema disease severity scales. Ophthalmology 2003;110:1677–82.

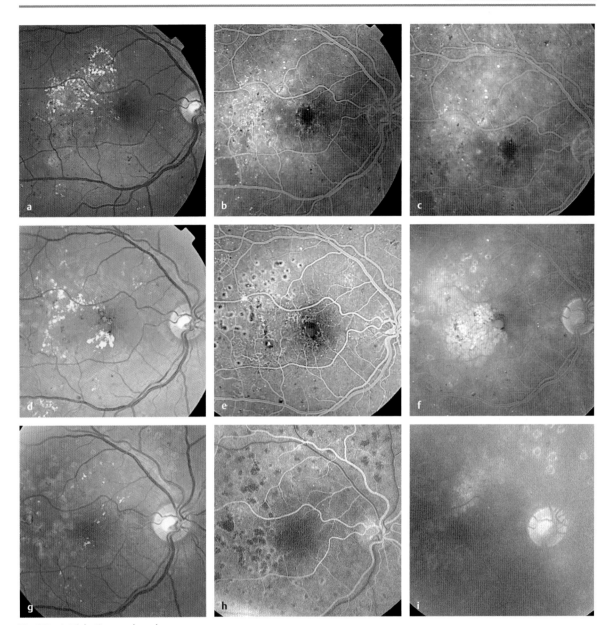

Fig. 6.2a–i Diabetic macular edema

a Color photograph. Focal diabetic macular edema. Hard exudates can be seen temporal and superior to the fovea.

b Early arteriovenous phase. Ectatic capillaries and micro-aneurysms, as well as localized areas with closed capillaries temporal and superior to the fovea, can be seen.

c Late phase. There is diffuse hyperfluorescence temporal and superior to the fovea in the area of the permeable capillaries. Focal paracentral laser coagulation has been carried out in the area of the hard exudates.

d Color photograph. Two years later, new hard exudates have appeared, extending from the temporal retina to the fovea. The exudates visible in a have disappeared after laser coagulation.

e Early arteriovenous phase. Laser scars in the area of the hard exudates shown in a. Rarefaction and ectatic changes of retinal capillaries can be seen temporal to the fovea. The parafoveal capillary arcades show discontinuity, a sign of initial central ischemia.

f Late phase. There is distinct hyperfluorescence with a cystoid component temporal to the fovea. Further paracentral focal laser coagulation has been carried out just temporal to the fovea.

g Color photograph. Two years later, the hard exudates shown in d have been resorbed after the additional laser coagulation. Some new, smaller hard exudates can be seen above the fovea.

h Early arteriovenous phase. Laser scars temporal to the fovea.

i Late phase. There is focal mild hyperfluorescence superior to the fovea, a sign of recurrent focal macular edema. Additional coagulation (focal and superior to the fovea) should be carried out in this case.

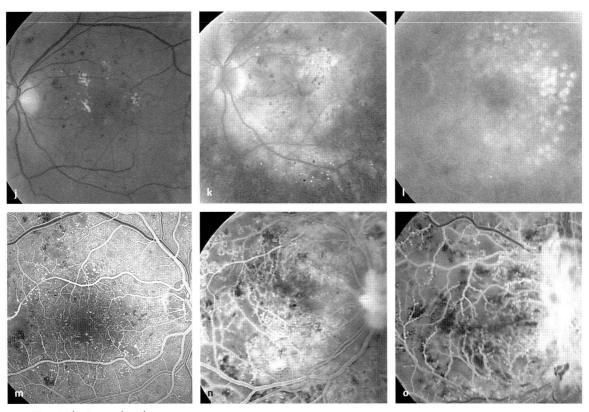

Fig. 6.2j–o Diabetic macular edema

j Color photograph. Diffuse diabetic macular edema. Some hard exudates and retinal hemorrhages can be seen paracentrally. Stereoscopic ophthalmoscopy shows swelling of the central retina, which is not visible in the two-dimensional picture.

k Late phase. Diffuse hyperfluorescence of the entire posterior pole due to diffuse capillary hyperpermeability.

l Late phase. Six months after paracentral grid laser coagulation, the diffuse capillary leakage and late hyperfluorescence have clearly diminished.

m Early arteriovenous phase (in a different patient). There is incipient ischemic maculopathy, with rarefaction of the juxtafoveal capillaries.

n Arteriovenous phase (in a different patient). There is significant central ischemia, with extensive capillary occlusion in the macula and ectatic deformations of the remaining capillaries. There is neovascularization on the optic nerve, evident from the increasing fluorescein leakage.

o Early arteriovenous phase (in a different patient). There is severe retinal ischemia, with almost complete occlusion of the capillaries; only the large arterioles are still perfused. A large proliferation can be seen on the optic nerve head, with fluorescein leakage.

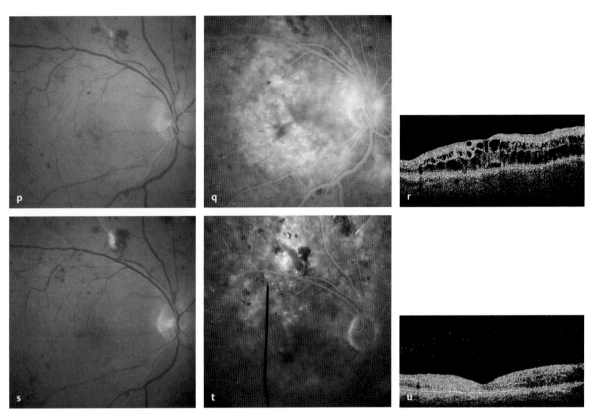

Fig. 6.**2p–u Diabetic macular edema**

p Color photograph. Diffuse diabetic macular edema, visual acuity was 0.05.

q Late phase. Extensive hyperfluorescence indicating severe cystoid macular edema.

r Optic coherence tomography (OCT). Marked thickening of the macula and cystoid spaces are visible.

s Color photograph (same patient as **p–r**). Six weeks after intravitreal injection of 4 mg triamcinolone acetonide. Visual acuity has improved to 0.25.

t Late phase. Regression of diffuse hyperfluorescence in the macula compared to **q**. Although a fixation needle is seen on the image, fixation was not maintained during this image.

u OCT picture. The paracentral retina is still a little thickened but the cystoid spaces have disappeared and the foveal impression is restored.

6

6.3 Proliferative Diabetic Retinopathy   *Horst Helbig*

Epidemiology, Pathophysiology, and Clinical Presentation

- Proliferative diabetic retinopathy occurs in approximately 45% of patients with type 1 diabetes after 20 years of diabetes, in less than 10% of those with type 2 diabetes not receiving insulin treatment, and in approximately 20% of those with type 2 diabetes receiving insulin treatment.
- The ischemic retina produces growth factors that stimulate neovascularization.
- The new vessels do not develop in the retina itself, but penetrate the inner limiting membrane, proliferate on the surface of the retina, or use the adjacent vitreous as a path for growth into the vitreous body.
- Neovascularization can be observed on the optic nerve head (new vessels on the disc, NVD), epiretinally (new vessels elsewhere, NVE), most often in the mid-periphery, or on the iris (rubeosis iridis).
- Complications that can lead to reduced visual acuity include vitreous hemorrhage, tractional retinal detachment, and neovascular glaucoma.

Fluorescein Angiography

- In contrast to normal retinal vessels, the new vessels have fenestrated vessel walls. Angiographically, they appear as increasingly indistinct areas of hyperfluorescence due to the effusion of dye.
- Preretinal neovascularization emerges mainly on the edge of the retinal areas affected by capillary occlusion.
- Optic disc proliferations occasionally fill earlier than the retinal vessels, suggesting a possible afferent supply of these vessels from the ciliary circulation.
- New vessels shrink after disseminated laser coagulation and become fibrotic, but usually do not disappear completely. In the late phase of fluorescein angiography, the residual connective tissue from treated proliferative vessels stains more weakly than actively proliferating vessels.

Diagnosis and Treatment

- The diagnosis and classification is based on the clinical examination. Angiography can confirm the presence of neovascularization in suspect areas.
- Treatment is carried out by ablating the ischemic retina using panretinal scatter laser coagulation. Approximately 20–40% of the peripheral retina is coagulated with disseminated laser spots, reducing the retina's consumption of oxygen and nutrients. This reduces the production of growth factors leading to retinal neovascularization.
- In difficult cases with rubeosis of the iris and/or media opacities, the peripheral retina can also be treated with cryotherapy.
- Vitrectomy can be carried out in cases of vitreous hemorrhage or tractional retinal detachment.

References

Diabetic Retinopathy Study Research Group. Photocoagulation treatment of proliferative diabetic retinopathy: clinical application of Diabetic Retinopathy Study (DRS) findings, DRS report number 8. Ophthalmology 1981;88:583–600.

Diabetic Retinopathy Vitrectomy Study Research Group. Early vitrectomy for severe vitreous hemorrhage in diabetic retinopathy: two-year results of a randomized trial. Diabetic Retinopathy Vitrectomy Study report 2. Arch Ophthalmol 1985;103:1644–52.

Ferris FL 3rd, Davis MD, Aiello LM. Treatment of diabetic retinopathy. N Engl J Med 1999;341:667–78.

Helbig H, Sutter FK. Surgical treatment of diabetic retinopathy. Graefes Arch Clin Exp Ophthalmol 2004;242:704–9.

6

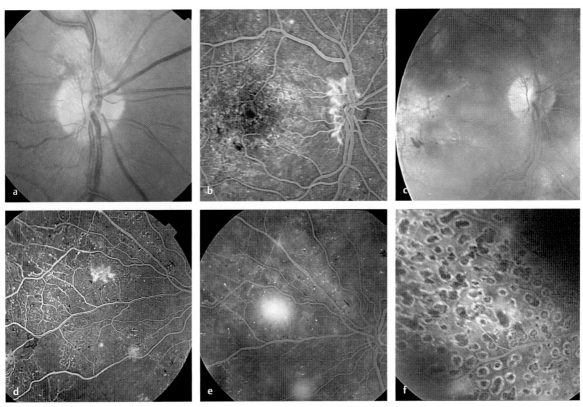

Fig. 6.3a–f Proliferative diabetic retinopathy

a Color photograph. Optic disc neovascularization.

b Middle arteriovenous phase. The optic disc proliferation is filling with dye. The fluorescein in the vessel lumen is leaking through the fenestrated vessel walls and is able to spread into the adjacent vitreous. As a result, the optic disc proliferation appears indistinct. Ectatic changes are present in the macular capillaries.

c Late phase. Dye has leaked into the vitreous body, and the image consequently appears indistinct, as if being seen through bright fog. The optic disc proliferation appears hypofluorescent, because the fluorescein has in the meantime been washed out of the vessel lumen. Diffuse macular edema with cystoid components can also be seen.

d Middle arteriovenous phase (in a different patient). There is preretinal proliferation in the mid-periphery, near areas with marked capillary occlusion.

e Late phase. Fluorescein has leaked into the area due to the permeable walls in the proliferative vessel, creating the appearance of a diffuse hyperfluorescent "cloud."

f Late phase. After scatter laser coagulation, the new vessel has regressed and undergone fibrosis. The fibrosis shows weak, diffuse staining in the late phase, but there is no evidence of any further active neovascularization.

6

7.1 Hypertensive Retinopathy

Heinrich Heimann

Epidemiology, Pathophysiology, and Clinical Presentation

- Diseases of the cardiovascular system are the most frequent causes of morbidity and mortality in the industrialized nations, and hypertension is the most important treatable risk factor for cardiovascular disease. In the USA, 38% of the population between 45–64 and 71% of the population of 65 years and over are affected.
- Hypertensive retinopathy can be observed with acute or chronic increases in blood pressure. It is an independent risk factor for increased cardiovascular mortality.
- In patients with chronic hypertension, focal narrowing of the arterioles, capillary hypoperfusion, and cotton-wool spots are seen. Damage to the blood–retina barrier, leading to intraretinal hemorrhage and exudates, can also be noted. Long-term changes in the vascular architecture lead to endothelial-cell hyperplasia, hyalinization of the intima, and hypertrophy of the media, which are visible ophthalmoscopically in the form of copper-wire arteries and can lead to signs of arteriovenous crossing. In extreme cases, the disease progresses to proliferative retinopathy and edema of the optic nerve head.
- When there are acute and massive increases in blood pressure, hypertensive choroidopathy may be observed. As a result of fibrinoid necrosis of the choroidal vessels, focal damage to the outer blood–retina barrier at the pigment epithelium takes place, with localized retinal detachment. Focal hyperpigmentation of the retinal pigment epithelium with a surrounding halo (Elschnig spots) can be seen in the healing phase.
- Patients with hypertensive retinopathy have an increased risk of developing retinal macroaneurysms (see section 7.7), retinal vein occlusions (see sections 7.3, 7.4), and anterior ischemic optic neuropathy (see section 10.1).
- Pregnancy-induced hypertension in preeclamptic patients induces retinal and choroidal ischemia that is usually diagnosed ophthalmoscopically.

Fluorescein Angiography

- The basic signs of hypertensive retinopathy can be diagnosed ophthalmoscopically, without angiography; however, advanced vessel changes can be visualized better using angiography.
- In advanced cases, retinal capillary occlusion (areas of hypofluorescence due to hypoperfusion), changes to the capillary architecture (particularly perifoveal, peripapillary, temporal to the fovea, and along the arterioles), microaneurysms (dot-like areas of increasing hyperfluorescence with moderate leakage), increased vessel tortuosity (particularly in the arterioles), arteriovenous anastomoses (new vessel lumina with low leakage) and leakage over the optic nerve head, in conjunction with optic disc swelling, can all be observed using fluorescein angiography.
- Choroidal filling is often delayed and irregular, and is sometimes only recognizable after filling of the retinal vessels has taken place.
- Focal leakages arise over pigment epithelial defects in hypertensive choroidopathy.

Diagnosis and Treatment

- Medical treatment for arterial hypertension is the initial measure. Visual acuity is often still surprisingly good in patients with hypertensive retinopathy, even in those with advanced disease.
- Ophthalmological diagnosis is clinically important when there is acute blood pressure deterioration (in patients with previously unknown hypertension), for identifying chronic retinal vessel changes in newly diagnosed hypertension, and in patients with advanced retinopathy. Ophthalmological treatment using laser coagulation is generally necessary if proliferative retinopathy develops.

References

Duncan BB, Wong TY, Tyroler HA, Davis CE, Fuchs FD. Hypertensive retinopathy and incident coronary heart disease in high risk men. Br J Ophthalmol 2002;86:1002–6.

Hayreh SS. Classification of hypertensive fundus changes and their order of appearance. Ophthalmologica 1989;198:247–60.

Klein R, Klein BE, Moss SE. The relation of systemic hypertension to changes in the retinal vasculature: the Beaver Dam Eye Study. Trans Am Ophthalmol Soc 1997;95:329–50.

Lafaut BA, De Vriese AS, Stulting AA. Fundus fluorescein angiography of patients with severe hypertensive nephropathy. Graefes Arch Clin Exp Ophthalmol 1997;235:749–54.

Pache M, Kube T, Wolf S, Kutschbach P. Do angiographic data support a detailed classification of hypertensive fundus changes? J Hum Hypertens 2002;16:405–10.

7

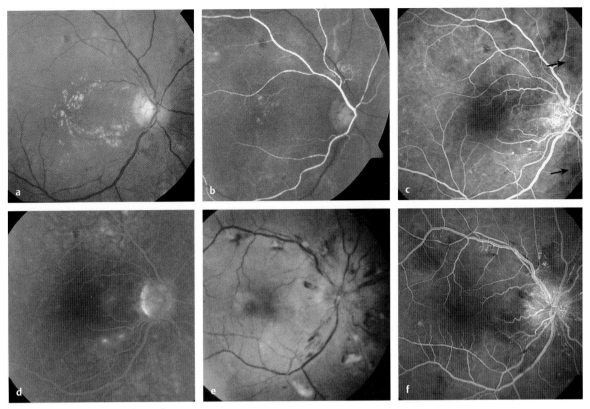

Fig. 7.1a–f Hypertensive retinopathy

a Color photograph. Star-shaped hard exudates are seen in the macula, as well as stenotic retinal arteries with thickened vessel walls, signs of arteriovenous crossing and collateral vessels, particularly below and above the optic nerve head.

b Arterial phase. Choroidal filling is delayed and segmented. The retinal arterioles show wall irregularities and are clearly constricted. Collateral vessels are visible above the optic nerve head. The hard exudates are sometimes not visible on fluorescence angiography and are only discernible as weak areas of hypofluorescence in the early phase. They cease to be visible during the course of the angiography.

c Arteriovenous phase. Collateral vessels can be seen above the optic nerve head, as abnormally directed vessel channels with only minimal leakage. Areas of hypofluorescence secondary to capillary occlusion (arrows) can be seen distal to the collateral vessels. Mild hypofluorescence due to the central retinal edema is visible in the fovea. The choroid still shows segmental, incomplete filling.

d Late phase. Two small vessel proliferations in the temporal lower vessel arcade can be identified due to preretinal leakage. The vascular anomalies close to the optic nerve head do not present a similar leakage phenomena in the late phase. Low-grade hyperfluorescence of the optic nerve head is visible.

e Color photograph. Hypertensive retinopathy, with narrowing of the retinal arteries, increased wall reflexes, arteriovenous crossing signs, cotton-wool spots, striped hemorrhage, and optic disc swelling.

f Arteriovenous phase. The cotton-wool spots are recognizable as discrete areas of hypofluorescence. Marked congestion and collateral hyperfluorescences can be seen on the optic disc. Speckled and delayed choroidal filling, capillary dropout and adjacent formation of collateral vessels above and below the optic disc, as well as in the temporal vessel arcade area, can be seen. The hemorrhage continues to be visible as constant, clear, and limited areas of hypofluorescence during the course of the angiography.

7

7.2 Ocular Ischemic Syndrome   *Heinrich Heimann*

Epidemiology, Pathophysiology, and Clinical Presentation

- In the ocular ischemic syndrome, retinal hypoperfusion takes place as a result of narrowing of the ipsilateral carotid artery (with narrowing of the lumen by more than 80%), mostly secondary to arteriosclerosis.
- Patients often report amaurosis fugax, or slow or sudden reductions in visual acuity; however, the disease can also become symptomatic without visual disturbances—for example, due to a secondary glaucoma. Ocular or periorbital pain is a relatively typical symptom (and is also independent of the appearance of a secondary glaucoma). The patients are usually over 60, with men being affected more often than women.
- The estimated incidence is between one in 10 000 and one in 100 000. The disease pattern is probably underdiagnosed and is frequently confused with other retinal vessel diseases. Bilateral disease is observed in approximately 20% of the patients.
- Neovascularization of the anterior segment occurs in 60–80% of the affected patients. Additional characteristics include a pale optic disc, constriction of the retinal arteries, distension of the veins, and fundus hemorrhages. Retinal neovascularization occurs in up to 13% of the patients.
- The syndrome is associated with diabetes mellitus (56%), hypertension (50%), coronary sclerosis (38%), and symptomatic cerebral hypoperfusion (31%). Patients with ocular ischemic syndrome have a markedly increased risk of other arterial occlusive diseases, such as cerebral and cardiac ischemia.

Fluorescein Angiography

- Typical findings are a delay in the appearance of fluorescein in the retinal/choroidal circulation system (with prolongation of the arm–retina time, which is normally 10–12 s) and an extended arteriovenous passage time.
- Irregular filling of the vascular system is also noticeable in addition to the delay during choroidal filling.
- The arteries are generally constricted and the veins distended, but venous beading is not usually seen.

- Dot hemorrhages (hypofluorescence due to blockages) and microaneurysms (increasing dot-shaped areas of hyperfluorescence) in the middle and distant periphery (and occasionally also at the posterior pole) can be distinguished angiographically. The hemorrhages are rarely confluent—a characteristic that distinguishes them from venous occlusions.
- Persistent fluorescence of the vessel walls of the retinal arteries in the late phase of angiography can be observed—in contrast to retinal arterial occlusion (in which there is no late fluorescence) or vein occlusion (which is particularly evident in the retinal veins).
- In a small proportion of affected patients, macular edema may be observed (with a late accumulation of hyperfluorescence in the macula without associated neovascularization).
- Angiographically, cotton-wool spots show moderate hypofluorescence due to localized hypoperfusion and blockage phenomena.

Diagnosis and Treatment

- Medical and neurological work-up, including an examination of the carotid arteries, should be carried out if ocular ischemic syndrome is suspected clinically.
- Retinal perfusion can be improved and a reduction in the reported ocular symptoms can be achieved in a number of patients by lumen extension or bypass surgery.
- Panretinal laser coagulation can lead to regression of the proliferative disease in areas of neovascularization.
- Generally, however, the prognosis with regard to the preservation of good visual acuity or a good peripheral field of vision is poor in clinically symptomatic patients.

References

Biousse V. Carotid disease and the eye. Curr Opin Ophthalmol 1997;8:16–26.

Brown GC, Magargal LE. The ocular ischemic syndrome: clinical, fluorescein angiographic and carotid angiographic features. Int Ophthalmol 1988;11:239–51.

Dugan JD Jr, Green WR. Ophthalmologic manifestations of carotid occlusive disease. Eye 1991;5:226–38.

Mizener JB, Podhajsky P, Hayreh SS. Ocular ischemic syndrome. Ophthalmology 1997;104:859–64.

7

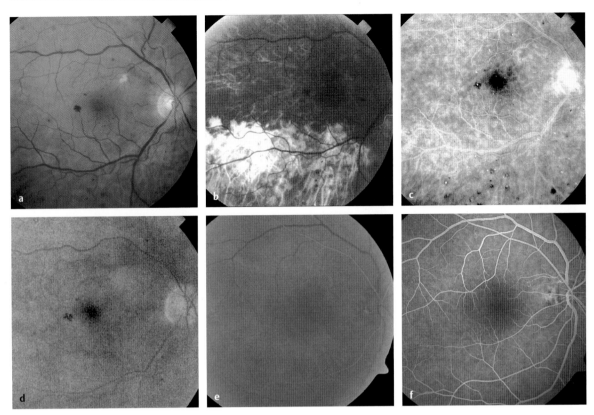

Fig. 7.2a–f Ocular ischemic syndrome

a Color photograph. Ocular ischemic syndrome in a patient with advanced carotid artery occlusion. The 58-year-old patient presented with a rubeosis of unclear etiology; his visual acuity had fallen to 0.5. Doppler ultrasonography demonstrated a high-grade ipsilateral occlusion in the carotid artery. Ophthalmoscopy shows disseminated, nonconfluent areas of hemorrhage, with microaneurysms and a cotton-wool spot. The veins are distended, with no evidence of venous beading. The arteries are narrowed.

b Early phase. After 15 s, there is clearly delayed, inhomogeneous choroidal filling. The retinal vessels are also filling with a definite delay.

c Arteriovenous phase. The time between the first appearance of the dye in the arteries and complete filling of the veins was over

20 s in this patient (normally up to 11 s). Dot-shaped hyperfluorescence in the region of the microaneurysms can be seen at the entire posterior pole, along with hyperfluorescence over the optic nerve head.

d Late phase. Mild macular edema and persistent blockage is visible due to the areas of hemorrhage.

e Arterial phase (in a different patient). Hypoperfusion in high-grade stenosis of the carotid arteries; the patient did not report any reduction in visual acuity. Very weak appearance of the dye in the retinal vessels can be seen only after 20 s.

f Arteriovenous phase. Again, more than 20 s pass before complete filling of the retinal veins. No areas of hemorrhage or microaneurysms are evident yet.

7

7.3 Central Retinal Vein Occlusion   *Heinrich Heimann*

Epidemiology, Pathophysiology, and Clinical Presentation

- Central retinal vein occlusion (CRVO) occurs as a result of thrombosis of the central retinal vein at the level of, and posterior to, the lamina cribrosa. Secondary to the occlusion, there is an increase in hydrostatic pressure, with extrusion of blood components from the retinal vessels and a clear deceleration of the retinal bloodstream. Risk factors include arterial hypertension, ocular hypertension, glaucoma, damage to the vascular wall (e. g., in diabetes mellitus and inflammatory conditions), and an increase in blood viscosity.
- Ophthalmoscopically, intraretinal and subretinal hemorrhages can be identified in all four quadrants, along with retinal edema with loss of retinal transparency, cotton-wool spots, extended and increased tortuosity of retinal veins, optic nerve head edema, and macular edema. The changes can appear with different grades of severity and with a wide range of interindividual variation.
- CRVO is usually classified as ischemic or nonischemic, but it should be borne in mind that definitions vary from study to study. Some 30 % of CRVOs are assigned to the ischemic form.
- Apart from the angiographic criteria, ischemic CRVO—in contrast to nonischemic CRVO—usually presents with a large number of fundus hemorrhages and cotton-wool spots, visual acuity of < 0.1, loss of peripheral visual fields, relative afferent pupillary deficit, and reduced amplitudes and delayed timing in the full-field electroretinogram.
- Major complications include a permanent reduction in visual acuity resulting from macular damage and the development of a neovascular glaucoma, which usually occurs within 7–8 months of the onset of the disease with ischemic CRVO.
- During the course of the disease, stages ranging from complete blindness to full recovery of visual acuity are possible. A permanent reduction in visual acuity occurs as a result of persistent macular edema, damage to either the perifoveal capillary network or the retinal pigment epithelium, prolonged retinal ischemia, or optic disc damage due to secondary glaucoma.
- The prevalence is 0.1 %, a rate that is approximately five times less than that of branch retinal vein occlusion. The risk of neovascular glaucoma developing is 30–50 % for ischemic CRVO and less than 10 % for nonischemic CRVO. The risk of contracting central retinal vein occlusion in the fellow eye is < 10 %.

Fluorescein Angiography

- The retinal veins appear broadened snake-like and have delayed filling in the venous phase of angiography. The arteriovenous time is usually prolonged. In severe cases, there is prolonged fluorescence of the vein walls.
- In the area of the occlusion, fleck-shaped and sometimes confluent intraretinal and preretinal hemorrhages (hypofluorescence due to blockage), retinal edema (hypofluorescence due to blockage), capillary occlusions or retinal ischemia (hypofluorescence due to hypoperfusion), intraretinal hard exudates, and cotton-wool spots can all be observed.
- In the late phase, areas of hyperfluorescence over the blocked veins due to dysfunction of the blood–retina barrier can be seen.
- Some of the natural papillary vein drainage takes place via cilioretinal vessels. In CRVO, these are visible in angiography as collaterals with increased filling, usually without significant leakage.
- Capillary occlusion in more than 10 disc diameters of the retinal surface (approximately 50 % of the retina in 30° exposures) can be used as a fluorescein-angiographic characteristic to distinguish between ischemic and nonischemic CRVO. However, this criterion is not appropriate as a single distinctive sign for distinguishing between the two disease groups, particularly since it can often not be assessed in the first few weeks of the disease (for example, in cases of extensive hemorrhage).
- Vascular anastomoses and anomalies (better visualized with fluorescein angiography, which usually shows no leakage or only slight leakage), telangiectases (irregular vessels with moderate hyperfluorescence), and vessel proliferations (hyperfluorescence from newly formed vessels, displaying clear leakage), along with secondary glaucoma and vitreous hemorrhage, can all develop in the course of the disease.

Diagnosis and Treatment

- More than 50 % of patients with nonischemic CRVO maintain or recover visual acuity of 0.5 or more during the natural course of the disease.
- The current treatment approaches (hemodilution, anticoagulant drug treatment, radial optic neurotomy, induction of retinochoroidal anastomoses by laser coagulation, and intravitreal corticosteroid injections) are controversial, and the results have not been confirmed in prospective multicenter studies.
- In macular edema, the amount of leakage visible in the angiogram can be reduced using central laser coagulation, but this does not lead to improved visual acuity.
- In ischemic CRVO, panretinal coagulation is recommended when areas of neovascularization appear in retina or in the iridocorneal angle. This is advocated as a preventive measure in ischemic CRVO by several groups, but it is highly controversial, since only just under half of the patients develop neovascular glaucoma and coagulation causes a reduction in the visual field.

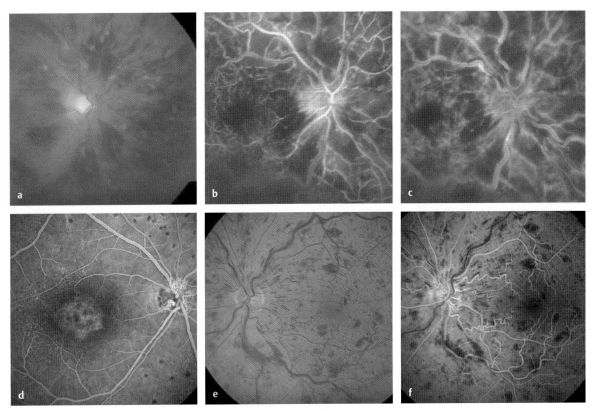

Fig. 7.**3a–f Central retinal vein occlusion**

a Color photograph. Ischemic central retinal vein occlusion, with massive retinal edema, cotton-wool spots, distended veins and increased tortuosity of the vessels, and disseminated retinal hemorrhages in all quadrants.

b Arteriovenous phase. There are areas of hypofluorescence due to hemorrhage (blockage) and extended capillary dropout (hypoperfusion), and areas of hyperfluorescence due to leakage from the distended vessels and accumulation in the vessel walls. There is a clearly extended arteriovenous passage time.

c Late arteriovenous phase. Increasing preretinal leakage is evident from the diffuse fluorescein leakage from the damaged vessels. Fluorescein staining is seen in the congested vein walls.

d Arteriovenous phase (in a different patient) 1 year after ischemic central retinal vein occlusion. Pigment epithelial changes in the central macula (with clearly demarcated areas of hyperfluores-

cence and hypofluorescence), capillary dropout and expansion of the parafoveal capillary network, and extended cilioretinal shunt vessels on the optic nerve head, are recognizable as sequelae of the central retinal vein occlusion. Scarred laser coagulation spots are visible above and below (a hypofluorescent center with a hyperfluorescent rim).

e Color photograph. Nonischemic central retinal vein occlusion with relatively few areas of streaky retinal hemorrhage, moderately extended veins with increased tortuosity, no cotton-wool spots, mild retinal edema, and low-grade macular edema.

f Arteriovenous phase. There is moderate distension and increased filling of the retinal veins, a moderately extended arteriovenous passage time, no capillary dropout, mild congestion with extended capillaries in the optic nerve head region, no leakage, and hypofluorescence due to hemorrhage (blockage).

References

Cooney MJ, Fekrat S, Finkelstein D. Current concepts in the management of central retinal vein occlusion. Curr Opin Ophthalmol 1998;9:47–50.

Hayreh SS. Management of central retinal vein occlusion. Ophthalmologica 2003;217:167–88.

Hayreh SS. Prevalent misconceptions about acute retinal vascular occlusive disorders Prog Retin Eye Res 2005;24:493–519.

Hayreh SS, Zimmerman MB, Podhajsky P. Hematologic abnormalities associated with various types of retinal vein occlusion. Graefes Arch Clin Exp Ophthalmol 2002;240:180–96.

7.4 Branch Retinal Vein Occlusion   *Heinrich Heimann*

Epidemiology, Pathophysiology, and Clinical Presentation

- After diabetic retinopathy, branch retinal vein occlusion (BRVO) is the second most common retinal vascular disease, with a prevalence of 0.6%. The risk of the fellow eye developing a vein occlusion is 10%.
- BRVO typically affects patients between 50 and 70 years of age and has no gender predilection. Arterial hypertension is a major risk factor.
- The pathophysiological mechanism is still unclear. Vessel wall damage and changes to the flow profile within the retinal vein probably play a decisive role.
- The occlusion develops distal to any crossing of arteries and veins, and the temporal quadrants are more regularly affected. An occlusion at the level of the optic nerve head leads to occlusion of half of the retina.
- There is a 40% risk of proliferative disease in the affected eye in an ischemic branch retinal vein occlusion (capillary nonperfusion over more than five disc diameters).
- BRVOs are generally symptomatic (with a sudden decrease in visual acuity or loss of visual fields). The reduced visual acuity is caused by macular edema, macular ischemia, or macular hemorrhage.

Fluorescein Angiography

- The affected venous branch is distended and shows delayed filling in the venous phase.
- Fleck-shaped, partly confluent areas of intraretinal and preretinal hemorrhage (hypofluorescence due to blockage), retinal edema (hypofluorescence due to blockage), capillary dropout with ischemia (hypofluorescence due to hypoperfusion), intraretinal hard exudates, and cotton-wool spots can all be observed in the area of the occlusion.
- In the late phase, hyperfluorescences are noticeable over the occluded vein and are typically also visible locally over the occlusion area.
- An important aspect for establishing the indication for laser coagulation is whether hyperfluorescence is visible in the late phase in the presence of macular edema, or whether the macular edema is ischemic (with extensive capillary dropout).
- In the course of the disease, vessel anastomoses develop and vessel anomalies occur (these are more visible with fluorescein angiography). Telangiectases

(irregular vessels with moderate hyperfluorescence), microaneurysms, and vessel proliferations (hyperfluorescence caused by newly formed vessels), with secondary glaucoma and vitreous hemorrhages, can also occur.
- In contrast to neovascularization, vessel collaterals do not show any fluorescein leakage.

Diagnosis and Treatment

- The diagnosis is generally reached from the typical clinical findings. Fluorescein angiography is indicated when there is a need to identify ischemic areas and leakage in patients with macular edema (rarely in the acute stage).
- The indications for laser treatment in macular edema are based on the Branch Vein Occlusion Study. Grid laser coagulation of the macula up to the vessel arcades should be carried out if there is visual acuity of 0.5 or less, and if leakage in the central macula is visible in the angiogram. Laser coagulation should not be carried out if the reduction in visual acuity is caused by hemorrhage or foveal ischemia.
- Laser coagulation in the ischemic area (at a distance of at least two disc diameters from the fovea) is indicated when there is evidence of neovascularization.
- Laser coagulation to prevent neovascularization in ischemic areas that are detectable with fluorescein angiography is a matter of controversy.
- Fluorescein angiography is not needed in extended intraretinal hemorrhage (acute stage). Resorption of the hemorrhage should be allowed to take place (as laser coagulation is not possible when there is extensive hemorrhage).

References

Christoffersen NL, Larsen M. Pathophysiology and hemodynamics of branch retinal vein occlusion. Ophthalmology 1999;106:2054–62.
Finkelstein D. Argon laser photocoagulation for macular edema in branch vein occlusion. Ophthalmology 1986;93:975–7.
Greaves M. Aging and the pathogenesis of retinal vein thrombosis. Br J Ophthalmol 1997;81:810–1.
Hayreh SS. Prevalent misconceptions about acute retinal vascular occlusive disorders Prog Retin Eye Res 2005;24:493–519.
Klein R, Klein BE, Moss SE, Meuer SM. The epidemiology of retinal vein occlusion: the Beaver Dam Eye Study. Trans Am Ophthalmol Soc 2000;98:133–41.

Fig. 7.4a–i Branch retinal vein occlusion

a Color photograph. Three months after branch retinal vein occlusion, areas of intraretinal hemorrhage, cotton-wool spots, and retinal edema are seen in the occlusion area. The affected vein shows increased tortuosity.

b Late arteriovenous phase. Hypofluorescence is visible in the occlusion area due to retinal edema and capillary dropout or destruction. Localized areas of hyperfluorescence caused by telangiectatic vessel changes can be seen.

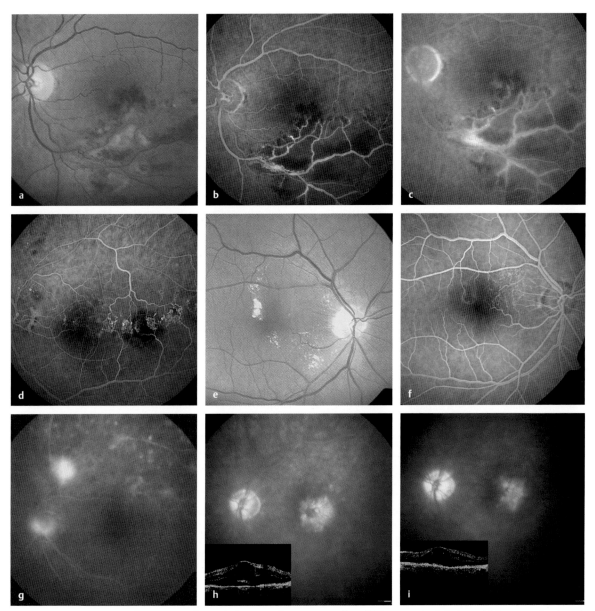

c Late phase. Areas of hyperfluorescence due to leakages in the macula and over the occlusion area can be seen. At the same time, areas of hypofluorescence resulting from hemorrhage extending to the fovea can still be seen. A further delay in laser treatment is therefore necessary. Laser coagulation should be considered after resorption of the hemorrhage and persistent leakage in the macula in patients with a visual acuity of 0.5 or less.

d Late arteriovenous phase (in a different patient). Several months after an occlusion of the temporal upper vein, numerous collaterals to the lower temporal arcade have developed. The collaterals are telangiectatic, distended, and show localized areas of hyperfluorescence.

e Color photograph. Persistent macular edema with hard exudates, several months after vein occlusion of the temporal upper arcade; the areas of hemorrhage have been completely resorbed.

f Arteriovenous phase. The development of telangiectatic vessels and collaterals can be seen. Laser photocoagulation should be considered if the late phases of the angiography (not shown here) demonstrate leakage in the central macula and the patient's visual acuity is less than 0.5.

g Late phase (different patient). Patient with long-standing branch retinal vein occlusion and neovascularizations on the disc and along the temporal superior vessel arcade. The neovascularizations are identifiable through late preretinal leakage over the proliferative vessels. No leakage is seen in the central macula. Therefore, photocoagulation outside the macula in the area of the venous occlusion should be performed. Previous laser spots are visible as hyperfluorescent spots with a hypofluorescent center in the superior temporal retinal quadrant.

h Late phase (different patient). Patient with long-standing cystoid macular edema secondary to branch retinal vein occlusion. Visual acuity had dropped to 0.1. Various therapeutic options were discussed with the patient and an intravitreal trimacinolone injection (4 mg) was performed, Inset: OCT demonstrating cystoid macular edema.

i Late phase (same patient as h). Only 4 weeks after the injection, visual acuity has improved to 0.4 and the patient regained reading ability. The late phase angiography and OCT (inset) show reduction of the cystoid macular edema. This therapy has not been supported by a prospective trial at the time of publication of this book.

7.5 Arterial Occlusion   *Heinrich Heimann*

Epidemiology, Pathophysiology, and Clinical Presentation

- Occlusion of the central retinal artery occurs at the level of the lamina cribrosa due to thrombus formation in arteriosclerosis, emboli, or inflammatory changes in the artery.
- The prevalence of retinal arterial emboli is 1%. The incidence of central arterial occlusion is reported to lie in the range of one in 10 000 to one in 100 000. Bilateral occlusions occur in 1–2% of cases. The majority of patients are over the age of 60, and men are affected more frequently.
- Occlusion occurs in the central artery in approximately 60% of patients and in the arterial branches in approximately 40%. Occlusion of the ophthalmic artery (occlusion of the retinal and choroidal circulation) can be observed in approximately 5% of cases.
- The clinical findings and the extent of the reduction in visual acuity depend on individual anatomy and the site of the occlusion (ophthalmic artery, central retinal artery, ciliary arteries, cilioretinal artery). A cilioretinal artery (a retinal vessel supplied by the ciliary arteries) may be found in up to 30% of patients; it may be either occluded or may remain patent when the central retinal artery is occluded, or it may be occluded independently.
- The clinical examination typically shows a relative afferent pupillary deficit. Ophthalmoscopically, the fundus findings may be inconspicuous during the first few hours; after this, increasing retinal edema appears in the inner retinal layers. A cherry-red spot in the macula is considered to be typical (with improved visibility of the retinal pigment epithelium and choroid through the fovea, in contrast to the surrounding edematous retina). In 20% of cases, intra-arterial emboli (e.g., cholesterol thrombi from the carotid arteries and fibrin–thrombocyte plaques from the cardiac valves) can be seen. During the course of the disease, reperfusion of the retinal vessels occurs, with thinning of the vascular lumina and of the retina and discoloration of the optic nerve head.
- Iris neovascularizations occur in 20% of patients, and optic nerve head proliferation appears in 5% of patients during the course of the disease.
- There is an association between arterial occlusion and hypertension (66%), diabetes mellitus (25%), diseases of the heart valves (25%), and temporal arteritis (2%). Patients with retinal arterial occlusions have a markedly increased risk of developing serious cardiovascular diseases (with arteriosclerotic changes).

Fluorescein Angiography

- The diagnosis can generally be established without angiography, on the basis of the typical clinical findings. However, fluorescein angiography may be helpful during first few hours of the occlusion in conditions in which the retinal edema is not yet particularly marked.
- Angiography cannot be expected to provide any significant additional information in clinically and ophthalmoscopically inconspicuous findings in patients with amaurosis fugax, with the exception of delayed choroidal and retinal filling in patients with ocular ischemic syndrome.
- Angiography shows a prolonged arm–retina time, prolonged filling of the retinal arteries, and a longer arteriovenous passage time, as well as late staining of the optic nerve head. In contrast to occlusions of the central retinal artery, choroidal filling is absent if the ophthalmic artery is affected (there is no background fluorescence). Perfusion of any cilioretinal vessels that may be present can be maintained and subsequently confirmed using fluorescein angiography.
- Intraluminal plaque formation, vessel wall changes, and changes in the flow profile can be visualized significantly better with angiography.
- Reperfusion of the arteries and a "normal" angiogram may be observed during the course of the disease. The vessels usually remain constricted.

Diagnosis and Treatment

- The patient usually notices a sudden, painless loss of visual acuity. Visual acuity of 0.5 or more is reached without treatment in 80–90% of patients with arterial branch occlusions or central arterial occlusions who have a patent cilioretinal artery. The disease is otherwise associated with a very bad prognosis regarding visual acuity (amaurosis or light perception).
- There are as yet no evidence-based approaches to treatment. Systemic or local thrombolytic therapy only appear to be promising in the first few hours after occlusion; however, the potential complications of this type of treatment in the group of patients affected also need to be taken into account. Other treatment approaches include anterior chamber tap or eyeball massage to reduce the intraocular pressure.

References

Duker JS, Sivalingam A, Brown GC, Reber R. A prospective study of acute central retinal artery obstruction: the incidence of secondary ocular neovascularization. Arch Ophthalmol 1991;109: 339–42.

Hayreh SS. Prevalent misconceptions about acute retinal vascular occlusive disorders. Prog Retin Eye Res 2005;24:493–519.

Ivanisevic M, Karelovic D. The incidence of central retinal artery occlusion in the district of Split, Croatia. Ophthalmologica 2001; 215:245–6.

Klein R, Klein BE, Jensen SC, Moss SE, Meuer SM. Retinal emboli and stroke: the Beaver Dam Eye Study. Arch Ophthalmol 1999;117: 1063–8.

Sharma S. The systemic evaluation of acute retinal artery occlusion. Curr Opin Ophthalmol 1998;9:1–5.

Wong TY, Klein R. Retinal arteriolar emboli: epidemiology and risk of stroke. Curr Opin Ophthalmol 2002;13:142–6.

7

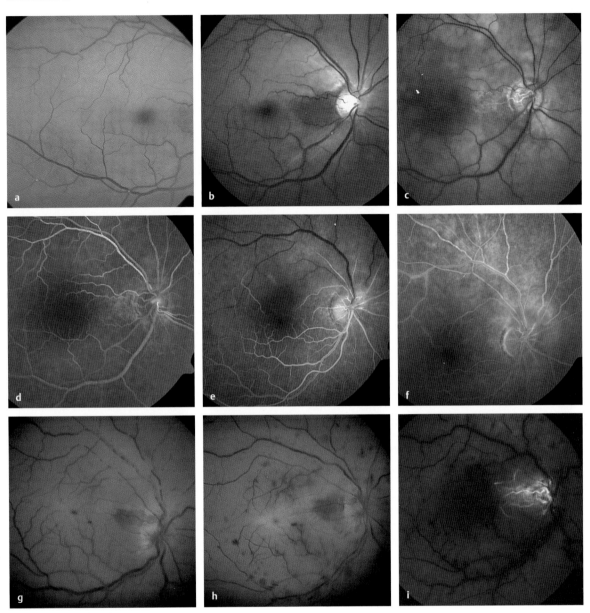

Fig. 7.**5a–i Arterial occlusion**

a Color photograph. Central retinal artery occlusion, with a cherry-red macular spot and multiple plaques in the upper and lower temporal arteries.

b Black-and-white photograph. There is retinal edema, with sparing of the papillomacular bundle.

c Arteriovenous phase. There is clearly delayed segmental choroidal filling. With the exception of a cilioretinal vessel, the retinal arteries have not filled. Drainage of the cilioretinal vessels via retinal veins above and below the papillomacular bundles can be seen.

d Late phase. After heavily delayed and low-grade perfusion of the retinal vessels, staining of the vessel walls (with fluorescein) and discrete leakage over the optic nerve head can be seen.

e Arteriovenous phase of an arterial occlusion of the upper hemisphere (in a different patient). The occluded arteries fill with a clearly reduced and broken column of blood, after a long delay.

f Late phase. The fluorescein from the vessels in the lower hemisphere has largely disappeared. In the upper hemisphere, persistent segmented staining of the vessel lumina of the veins takes place due to the reduced perfusion.

g Color photograph. Male patient with a sudden loss in visual acuity in the right eye. The picture shows a cherry-red spot in the fovea, surrounding retinal edema, segmented blood columns in the arteries and a small patch of non-edematous retina in the papillomacular bundle adjacent to the optic disc.

h Color photograph (same patient as in **g**). One day later, disseminated retinal hemorrhages can be seen in all retinal quadrants. This is a rather unusual finding in central retinal artery occlusions and points towards a possible vasculitic etiology of the vaso-occlusive disease. Medical workup established the diagnosis of Behçet disease (see section 9.2).

i Arteriovenous phase. Only a small cilioretinal artery remains perfused, explaining the patch of non-edematous retina adjacent to the optic disc.

7.6 Purtscher Retinopathy   *Andreas Schueler*

Epidemiology, Pathophysiology, and Clinical Presentation

- Purtscher retinopathy typically appears in an acute form after skull–brain trauma, chest injuries, and fractures of long bones in the extremities. An identical disease pattern can be seen in acute pancreatitis, lupus erythematodes, thrombocytopenic purpura, chronic renal failure, renal graft rejection, systemic autoimmune diseases, and coil embolization of intracranial carotid aneurysms.
- It has been speculated that intravascular microparticles (lipids, thrombocyte/leukocyte aggregates, and air embolism) may lead to the occlusion of peripapillary capillaries.
- Sudden loss of visual acuity, usually bilaterally, is the presenting symptom in the majority of patients.
- Clinically, confluent cotton-wool spots and retinal areas with superficial whitening of the retina at the posterior pole and around the optic nerve head are present; spot hemorrhages can occasionally also be seen.
- Edema of the optic nerve head may develop during the course of the disease, but does not form part of the initial clinical picture. Venous congestion with tortuosity can also develop as a secondary finding.
- In the majority of cases the peripheral retina is not affected.

Fluorescein Angiography

- Occlusion of small vessels (arterial branches) and capillaries is observed in the form of peripapillary hypofluorescence. The walls of the occluded vessels or of the efferent veins may show increased staining in the course of the disease.
- Dot-shaped areas of hyperfluorescence can appear adjacent to the cotton-wool spots in the late arteriovenous phase, continuing up to the late phase; if there is any hemorrhage, corresponding blockages of the background fluorescence can be observed.
- Hyperfluorescence of the optic nerve head in middle and late phases may appear in patients with secondary edema of the optic nerve head.

Diagnosis and Treatment

- The diagnosis can be made in patients with a known history of trauma and the typical clinical picture. A thorough medical examination should be carried out if the clinical findings appear with no history of trauma. Acute pancreatitis and vasculitic diseases are other conditions that have been associated with Purtscher retinopathy.
- Purtscher retinopathy is thought to be caused by acute embolic incidents, and there is no proven causative treatment for the previous injuries.
- When the cause is not traumatic, treatment of the etiogenic disease should be initiated.
- Cotton-wool spots and hemorrhages disappear within a few weeks. The prognosis for visual acuity depends entirely on the extent of the macular ischemia and the developing optic atrophy.

References

Behrens-Baumann W, Scheurer G, Schroer H. Pathogenesis of Purtscher's retinopathy. Graefes Arch Clin Exp Ophthalmol 1992;230: 286–91.

Gass JD. Obstructive retinal arterial disease. In: Gass JD, ed. Stereoscopic atlas of macular diseases: diagnosis and treatment, 4th ed. St. Louis: Mosby, 1997: 444–66.

Regillo CD, Brown GC, Flynn HW Jr. Vitreoretinal disease: the essentials. New York: Thieme, 1999:537–9.

7

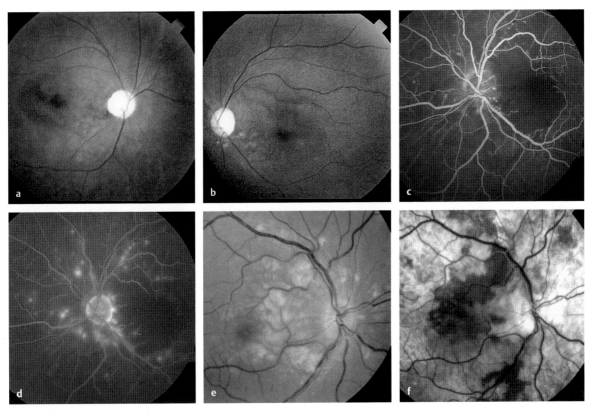

Fig. 7.6a–f Purtscher retinopathy

a Color photograph. Right eye with optic atrophy, juxtapapillary whitish retinal areas, and macular pigment clumping. The choriocapillaris also appears to be altered.

b Color photograph. There is an almost symmetrical development in the fellow eye. The patient was suffering from acute pancreatitis and had experienced a massive acute decrease in visual acuity some weeks before the examination.

c Middle arteriovenous phase. Macular hypofluorescence (arterial branch occlusion, capillary occlusions in the retina and choroid) and focal dot-shaped spots of hyperfluorescence on the edge of the ischemic areas. The walls of the occluded retinal vessels and the efferent veins are partly staining.

d Late phase. There is an increase in the areas of focal hyperfluorescence due to leakage phenomena. With optic atrophy, strong demarcation of the optic nerve head is seen.

e Color photograph. Purtscher retinopathy with cotton-wool spots at the posterior pole surrounding the optic nerve head, following chest trauma.

f Early phase. Delayed choroid filling with irregular fluorescence as a sign of a partial occlusion not only of the retinal vessels, but also of the choroid vessels. The retinal vessels are also clearly filling with a delay.

7

7.7 Retinal Arteriolar Macroaneurysms   *Andreas Schueler*

Epidemiology, Pathophysiology, and Clinical Presentation

- Arteriolar macroaneurysms typically appear in patients with arterial hypertension ($> 75\%$ of cases) and in the sixth or seventh decades of life. Women are affected much more often than men. Bilateral disease can be seen in 10% of cases.
- The majority of macroaneurysms appear in the temporal upper arterial branches, and they are almost always located central to the equator. Sites of predilection include arteriovenous crossings and vessel divisions.
- Damage to the dilated vessel wall leads to local leakage with surrounding retinal edema and circinate lipid exudates.
- Hemorrhage is observed in approximately 50% of cases. Subretinal and epiretinal hemorrhage suggests the diagnosis. Acute loss of visual acuity resulting from arteriolar macroaneurysm is often the first sign that leads to the diagnosis. Without accompanying hemorrhage or exudations, macroaneurysms are generally asymptomatic. Recurrent hemorrhage from macroaneurysms is rare.

Fluorescein Angiography

- In view of the clinical variability of the disease pattern, the fluorescein-angiographic findings can also be variable.
- Clearly demarcated areas of focal hyperfluorescence associated with vessels can already be seen in arteriolar macroaneurysms in the early phase of angiography. An absence of hyperfluorescence in cases in which an aneurysm is visible clinically suggests spontaneous thrombosis.
- In subretinal hemorrhage, a surrounding blockage of the background fluorescence can develop, while epiretinal hemorrhage can obscure the macroaneurysm.
- Surrounding hyperfluorescence can suggest focal exudation in the arteriovenous and late phases of angiography.

Diagnosis and Treatment

- The typical picture of a solitary circinate lipid exudation with centrally situated arteriolar vessel anomalies suggests the diagnosis. The diagnosis of secondary venous vessel changes and macroaneurysms—for example, after branch retinal vein occlusion or diabetic retinopathy—can be differentiated using fluorescein angiography.
- Retinal angiomas can usually be distinguished from macroaneurysms in von Hippel–Lindau syndrome by the typically dilated efferent and afferent vessels.
- Cavernous retinal hemangiomas are another differential diagnosis. They are often peripherally located, almost never show exudations, and are recognizable by their typical grape-shaped arrangement of the vascular malformations (Fig. 7.**7e**, **f**).
- A suspicion of macroaneurysm is raised if an epiretinal or subretinal juxtamacular hemorrhage is present at the posterior pole. The diagnosis can be obscured by the hemorrhage. In cases of massive vitreous hemorrhage with no recognizable cause, vitrectomy can be considered, and it may only be possible to diagnose a macroaneurysm intraoperatively.
- In patients with a solitary macular subretinal hemorrhage, the differential diagnosis has to include choroidal neovascularization in age-related macular degeneration.
- The treatment of arteriolar macroaneurysms varies. Spontaneous cures in the context of thrombosis are common. Follow-up examinations can therefore be considered if visual acuity is good and only mild exudation is observed. After massive subretinal hemorrhage with a poor prognosis for visual acuity, only surgery can be considered in addition to follow-up of the spontaneous course of the disease.
- Laser coagulation can be considered in patients with documented visual loss, increasing exudation threatening the macula, or recurrent hemorrhage. Laser treatment can either be carried out directly on the aneurysm or can be performed in the form of grid laser coagulation surrounding the aneurysm.
- The value of surgical procedures (such as vitrectomy [except for vitreous hemorrhage] intravitreal recombinant tissue plasminogen activator treatment, or gas injection) is still unclear at present.
- A thorough medical examination should be carried out in all patients with arteriolar macroaneurysms, in view of the high probability of arterial hypertension.

References

Brown DM, Sobol WM, Folk JC, Weingeist TA. Retinal arteriolar macroaneurysms: long-term visual outcome. Br J Ophthalmol 1994; 78:534–8.

Gass JD. Acquired retinal arterial macroaneurysms. In: Gass JD, ed. Stereoscopic atlas of macular diseases: diagnosis and treatment, 4th ed. St. Louis: Mosby, 1997: 472–6.

Humayun M, Lewis H, Flynn HW Jr, Sternberg P Jr, Blumenkranz MS. Management of submacular hemorrhage associated with retinal arterial macroaneurysms. Am J Ophthalmol 1998;126:358–61.

Kokame GT. Vitreous hemorrhage after intravitreal tissue plasminogen activator (t-PA) and pneumatic displacement of submacular hemorrhage. Am J Ophthalmol 2000;129:546–7.

Moosavi RA, Fong KC, Chopdar A. Retinal artery macroaneurysms: clinical and fluorescein angiographic features in 34 patients. Eye 2005 [epub ahead of print].

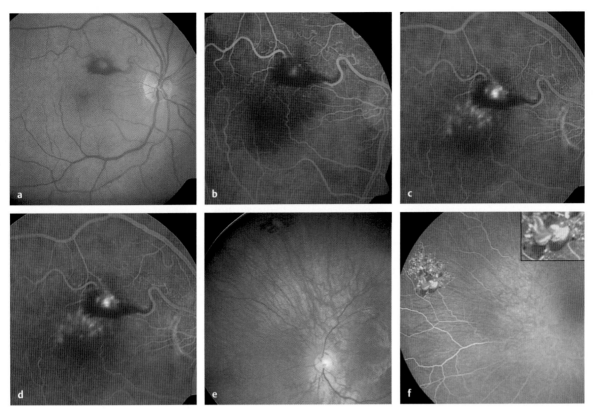

Fig. 7.**7a–f Retinal arteriolar macroaneurysms**

a Color photograph. A patient with a deterioration in visual acuity due to a retinal arteriolar macroaneurysm, with surrounding hemorrhage and retinal edema.

b Early phase. There is blockage in the area of the epiretinal hemorrhage, with central hyperfluorescence in the area of the aneurysm, the location of which is clearly associated with the retinal arteries.

c Middle arteriovenous phase. There is increasing hyperfluorescence in the aneurysm area and the development of diffuse enhancement in the area of the macula, as a cause of the decrease in visual acuity.

d Late phase. There is no significant further increase in the macular leakage. Spontaneous thrombosis of the aneurysm is clearly not evident. In this case, grid laser coagulation around the aneurysm could lead to improvement in the retinal edema.

e Color photograph. A cavernous retinal hemangioma with typical grape-shaped arrangement of the vessel dilations and malformations has to be considered in the differential diagnosis. This hereditary vessel anomaly is rarely associated with exudative changes if it is in a central position.

f Late phase. Protracted filling of the caverns without local exudation is characteristic. There is typical localized hyperfluorescence only in the upper half of the large vessel caverns (the lower half remains dark due to the sedimented erythrocytes). The inset shows magnification.

7

7.8 Coats Disease   *Andreas Schueler*

Epidemiology, Pathophysiology, and Clinical Presentation

- This rare disease of the retinal vessels represents the most important differential diagnosis against retinoblastoma. The cause is still unknown.
- Coats disease almost always appears in patients under the age of 10; in over 90% of cases, the condition is unilateral. Boys are more frequently affected than girls.
- The principal clinical symptoms are a decrease in visual acuity, leukokoria, heterochromy, secondary glaucoma, and pain.
- Typically, a peripheral retinal vessel anomaly with microaneurysms and capillary ectasia is observed.
- A defective endothelial lining in the vessels leads to a distinct exudation that can progress to a highly bullous retinal detachment.
- Intraretinal and subretinal exudates can be observed at the posterior pole and peripherally, with findings ranging up to subretinal lipid and cholesterol deposits that resemble pseudotumor (differential diagnosis: retinoblastoma).
- The vitreous cavity can also be affected if there is hemorrhage.
- Capillary occlusion leads to the development of ischemic retinopathy, which can progress up to the development of a painful neovascular secondary glaucoma.
- In retinitis pigmentosa, mid-peripheral vessel abnormalities resembling Coats disease may develop, often in association with mutations in the *CRB1* gene. Coats disease without retinitis pigmentosa is usually not associated with mutations in the *CRB1* gene.
- In some cases, peripheral Coats disease is associated with parafoveal telangiectasia (see section 7.10).

Fluorescein Angiography

- Fluorescein angiography is of little value for the differential diagnosis, particularly since the peripheral location of the changes can only rarely be adequately imaged in very young patients.
- Relatively slow filling of the peripheral capillary changes can be seen in the early phase. In addition, early blockage in the area of the subretinal lipid exudate can be observed.
- Clear demarcation of the area of capillary occlusion can be seen in the arteriovenous phase, as well as increasing filling of the aneurysms and capillary ectasia.

- Increasing and sometimes focal exudation occurs in the area of the vessel anomalies in the late arteriovenous phase.
- Diffuse hyperfluorescence from a massive subretinal accumulation of dye in the affected sector can be seen in the late phase.
- For clinical purposes, it is important to identify the exudation areas and ischemic zones.

Diagnosis and Treatment

- The diagnosis is based on the typical clinical appearance, excluding the possibility of a retinoblastoma. In patients with advanced exudative retinal detachments, additional radiographic examinations such as computed tomography and magnetic resonance imaging may be necessary.
- The goal of treatment is regression of the exudative vascular anomalies, as well as treatment of existing areas of capillary occlusion in order to prevent secondary complications.
- Laser coagulation therapy or cryotherapy can be carried out if early diagnosis has been achieved. Even after successful coagulation, regression of lipid exudates may take a long period of time, however.
- Vitrectomy with laser or cryo-endocoagulation should be considered in patients with existing bullous retinal detachments. It has been suggested that subretinal exudates can be removed via a retinotomy.
- Enucleation should be considered in patients with functional blindness and pain symptoms, or if it is not possible to rule out retinoblastoma conclusively.

References

Gass JD. Retinal capillary diseases. In: Gass JD, ed. Stereoscopic atlas of macular diseases: diagnosis and treatment, 4th ed. St. Louis: Mosby, 1997:476–515

Krause L, Kreusel KM, Jandeck C, Kellner U, Foerster MH. Vitrektomie bei fortgeschrittenem Morbus Coats. Ophthalmologe 2001;98: 387–90.

Moore A. Congenital and vascular abnormalities of the retina. In: Taylor D. Pediatric ophthalmology, 2nd ed. Boston: Blackwell, 1997:421–3.

Nucci P, Bandello F, Serafino M, Wilson ME. Selective photocoagulation in Coats' disease: ten-year follow-up. Eur J Ophthalmol 2002;12:501–5.

Shields JA, Shields CL, Honavar SG, Demirci H, Cater J. Classification and management of Coats disease: the 2000 Proctor Lecture. Am J Ophthalmol 2001;131:572–83.

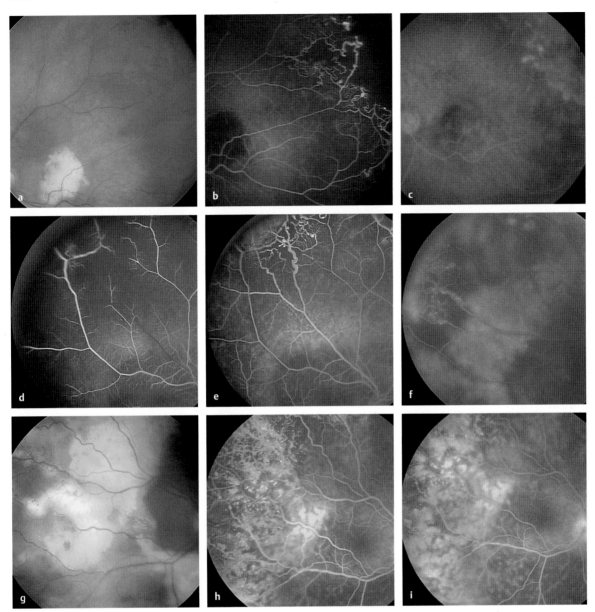

Fig. 7.8a–i Coats disease

a Color photograph. A 120° wide-angle exposure showing early-stage Coats disease. Peripheral capillary ectasia and typical subretinal lipid exudates can be seen, accumulated at the posterior pole.

b Early phase. There is slow filling of the dilated vessel anomalies. Initially, moderately leaking vessel ectasias with baggy or light-bulb-shaped extended vessel sections and aneurysms (areas of hyperfluorescence) can be seen in the region bordering the unperfused areas of the peripheral retina (hypofluorescence).

c Late arteriovenous phase. There is increasing diffuse hyperfluorescence due to the leaking vessels.

d Early phase (in a different patient). Slow filling of the dilated vessel anomalies, as well as blockages in the area of the lipid exudates at the posterior pole, can be seen.

e Middle arteriovenous phase. There is increasing filling of the aneurysms and the baggy extended vessel ectasias with adjoining capillary occlusion areas and incipient hyperfluorescence due to exudation.

f Late phase. There is massive diffuse hyperfluorescence due to areas of focal exudation in the region of the vessel anomalies.

g Color photograph. A 120° wide-angle exposure showing advanced Coats disease. There is a retinal detachment and diffuse subretinal lipid exudates due to peripheral capillary ectasias.

h Middle arteriovenous phase. There is increasing filling of the aneurysms and of the baggy extended vessel ectasias, with adjoining capillary occlusion areas and incipient hyperfluorescence due to exudations.

i Late phase. Massive diffuse hyperfluorescence is seen, due to focal exudation areas in the region of the vessel anomalies.

7.9 Eales Disease   *Andreas Schueler*

Epidemiology, Pathophysiology, and Clinical Presentation

- Eales disease is characterized by the development of peripheral obliterative vasculitis, with vessel sheathing and vessel occlusion. Patients are in usually in their 30s or 40s, and men are affected more often than women. The disease is especially common in Asia and in the Indian subcontinent. Bilateral involvement is observed in 80–90% of cases.
- The pathogenesis of Eales disease is not clear. A suspected connection with exposure to tuberculin antigens has not yet been demonstrated.
- Secondary inflammatory changes (endothelial precipitates, vitreitis, and macular edema) can be seen in the anterior and posterior segments.
- Typically, neovascularization or microvascular anomalies at the edge of a vascularized and peripheral ischemic retina appear in up to 80% of cases.
- Reduced visual acuity is caused by vitreous clouding or by cystoid macular edema.
- If the condition is left untreated, vitreous hemorrhage or a tractional retinal detachment can develop secondary to the neovascular proliferations.

Fluorescein Angiography

- Peripheral nonperfused retinal areas, with vessel anomalies at the border between still vascularized and ischemic retina, are important, but not pathognomonic, fluorescein-angiographic findings.
- In mild conditions, capillary ectasias can be seen at the edge of the hypofluorescent ischemic retina in the early phase. Extensive proliferations described as resembling a sea fan (a type of coral) can be seen when the disease is more fully developed. In the middle and late arteriovenous phases, these vascular anomalies can show increasing hyperfluorescence due to leakage. Hemor-

rhage from the pathological vessels leads to focal blockage of the background fluorescence.
- Typical fluorescein-angiographic findings also include macular and juxtamacular telangiectasia with cystoid macular edema in the late phase.

Diagnosis and Treatment

- Eales disease is a diagnosis of exclusion; it can only be established if no other signs of systemic disease are present that could lead to similar changes and symptoms (e. g., sickle-cell anemia, diabetic retinopathy, familial exudative vitreoretinopathy, sarcoidosis, collagenosis).
- The inflammatory components of the disease may respond to corticosteroid therapy.
- Laser coagulation or cryotherapy of the peripheral ischemic retina leads to regression of the proliferation and is used as the initial treatment of the disease.
- Vitrectomy is advisable if the disease course is complicated by vitreous hemorrhage, tractional retinal detachment, or secondary epiretinal gliosis.

References

Biswas J, Sharma T, Gopal L, Madhavan HN, Sulochana KN, Ramakrishnan S. Eales disease: an update. Surv Ophthalmol 2002;47: 197–214.

El-Asrar AM, Al-Kharashi SA. Full panretinal photocoagulation and early vitrectomy improve prognosis of retinal vasculitis associated with tuberculoprotein hypersensitivity (Eales' disease). Br J Ophthalmol 2002;86:1248–51.

Gass JD. Primary retinal vasculitis or vasculopathy (Eales' disease). In: Gass JD, ed. Stereoscopic atlas of macular diseases: diagnosis and treatment, 4th ed. St. Louis: Mosby, 1997: 534–8.

Mandava N, Yannuzzi LA. Miscellaneous Retinal Vascular Conditions. In: Regillo CD, Brown GC, Flynn HW Jr, eds. Vitreoretinal disease: the essentials. New York: Thieme, 1999: 202–4.

Shanmugam MP, Badrinath SS, Gopal L, Sharma T. Long term visual results of vitrectomy for Eales disease complications. Int Ophthalmol 1998;22:61–4.

7

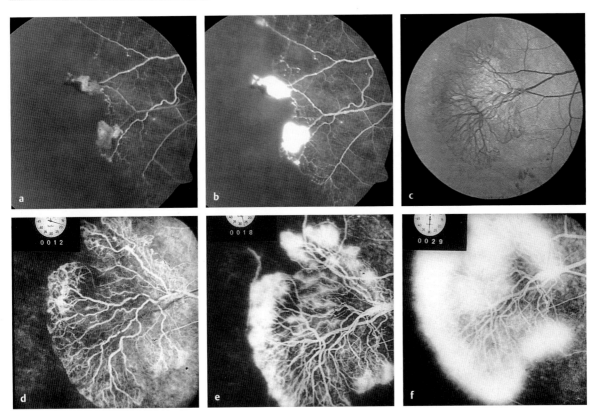

Fig. 7.9a–f Eales disease

a Early phase. Eales disease with peripheral ischemic retina. Capillary ectasias of the retinal vessels and neovascularization at the border of the ischemic retina can be seen.

b Late arteriovenous phase. There is leakage from the neovascularizations and complete ischemia of the peripheral retina.

c Color photograph. There is a marked "sea fan" neovascularization pattern on the border with the ischemic peripheral retina.

d Early phase. The neovascularization is clearly visible in the early arterial phase. Complete capillary and vessel dropout in the peripheral retina can be seen.

e Arteriovenous phase; transition to the middle arteriovenous phase. Areas of hyperfluorescence due to extended leakage from the newly formed vessels can be seen, as well as persistent hypofluorescence (ischemia) in the peripheral retina.

f Late arteriovenous phase. The continued increase in the leakage leads to massive hyperfluorescence in the area of neovascularization. In comparison with telangiectases, neovascularizations show significantly more leakage phenomena.

7

7.10 Parafoveal Retinal Telangiectasia   *Werner Inhoffen*

Epidemiology, Pathophysiology, and Clinical Presentation

- Telangiectases are irregularly broadened capillaries, which can progress to become large aneurysms. Histologically, they show thickening of the vessel wall and degeneration of pericytes. At the posterior pole, they are mostly located temporal to the fovea and display vascular occlusion, leakage, and tissue loss. The cause of the disease is unclear, and there are no reliable data regarding its prevalence or incidence.
- The condition may occur either with or without involvement of the peripheral retina. Coats disease is often present in patients with peripheral involvement (see section 7.8).
- Telangiectases without involvement of the retinal periphery are divided into the following subgroups in accordance with the Gass classification.
- Unilateral juxtafoveal telangiectasis (UJT), also known as idiopathic parafoveal telangiectasis (IPT). This group is further subdivided into:
  - Group 1A: congenital juxtafoveal retinal telangiectasis. This mainly affects men aged around 40 and is usually unilateral. Visible angiectases are found temporal to the fovea in an area at least one disc diameter wide, sometimes also with hard exudates and/or cystoid macular edema. Patients initially present with a visual acuity of approximately 0.5. Prognosis: slow decrease in vision. Treatment: laser photocoagulation can be attempted (coagulation of aneurysms or scatter).
  - Group 1B: congenital juxtafoveal retinal telangiectasis (rare). As in group 1A, the aneurysms do not extend far (about 2 clock hours juxtafoveally), but they reach the avascular zone. Laser coagulation is not recommended in these cases.
- Group 2: bilateral idiopathic juxtafoveal telangiectasis (BJT). These aneurysms show no gender predilection and are bilateral and initially occult on ophthalmoscopy. They are mostly located temporal to the fovea, without hard exudates. This type is less frequent than type 1A, and the patients initially present between 50 and 60 years of age. Prognosis: profound but slow decrease in vision; choroidal neovascularization or atrophy may develop.
- The different stages of the disease in the Gass classification are:
  1. No ophthalmoscopically visible changes; mild staining on angiography.
  2. Light gray discoloration on ophthalmoscopy; there may be yellow deposits, with only slight telangiectatic changes on angiography.
  3. Ophthalmoscopically visible capillary dilations.
  4. Ophthalmoscopically visible pigment clumping and chorioretinal anastomoses.
  5. Ophthalmoscopy and angiography show fibrovascular mass.
- Secondary telangiectasis can be seen in vein occlusion, diabetic retinopathy, hypertensive retinopathy, and radiation retinopathy. Polypoidal choroidal vasculopathy can be difficult to differentiate from telangiectasia; indocyanine green angiography is recommended in these cases (see section 3.10).

Fluorescein Angiography

- The telangiectatic vessel dilations already fill in the early phase. In contrast to neovascularizations, they usually display only moderate, but increasing leakage during angiography. When viewed stereoscopically, the leakage is seen to be located in the retina layer, in contrast to the leakage from neovascularizations. Vessel rarefaction can also be seen, and (in patients with adult Coats disease) additional vascular occlusion and aneurysms of the capillary bed can occur peripherally.
- In the late phase, there is diffuse leakage, centrally located (or also peripherally in adult Coats disease). In bilateral idiopathic juxtafoveal telangiectasis (BJT), fluorescein angiography provides specific findings, with minor, slow leakage and staining of the intraretinal cells, without pronounced edema.

Diagnosis and Treatment

- The individual subgroups can be distinguished using ophthalmoscopy and angiography.
- In unilateral juxtafoveal telangiectasis (type A UJT), perifoveal focal laser treatment is only indicated in the early stages. Laser coagulation is not recommended in type B UJT or bilateral idiopathic juxtafoveal telangiectasis (BJT). Experimental treatments have been carried out with photodynamic therapy and surgical procedures (vitrectomy or intravitreal corticosteroid injection) in patients with stage 5 BJT.

References

Barile GR, Yannuzzi L. Parafoveal telangiectasis. In: Guyer DR, Yannuzzi LA, Chang S, Shields JA, Green WR, eds. Retina–vitreous–macula. London: Saunders, 1999: 398–406.

Gass JD, Blodi BA. Idiopathic juxtafoveolar retinal telangiectasis: update of classification and follow-up study. Ophthalmology 1993;100:1536–46.

Haller JA. Coats' disease and retinal telangiectasis. In: Yanoff M, Duker JS, eds. Ophthalmology. London: Mosby, 2nd ed., 2004:896–901.

Park DW, Schatz H, McDonald HR, Johnson RN. Grid laser photocoagulation for macular edema in bilateral juxtafoveal telangiectasis. Ophthalmology 1997;104:1838–46.

Potter MJ, Szabo SM, Chan EY, Morris AH. Photodynamic therapy of a subretinal neovascular membrane in type 2A idiopathic juxtafoveolar retinal telangiectasis. Am J Ophthalmol 2002;133:149–51.

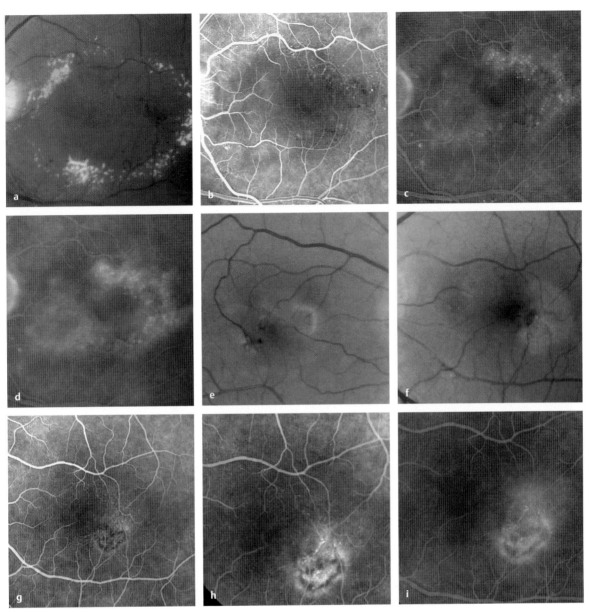

Fig. 7.10a–i Parafoveal retinal telangiectasia

a Color photograph. Central telangiectases in adult Coats disease. Hard exudates, macular edema, and visible aneurysms temporal to the fovea can be sen.

b Arteriovenous phase. Aneurysms and capillary occlusion can be seen; the hard exudates are only recognizable as weak, hypofluorescent areas in the angiogram.

c Late arteriovenous phase. There is leakage from the aneurysms and affected capillaries.

d Late phase. Further increase in the leakage is seen.

e Color photograph in a patient with stage 5 bilateral idiopathic juxtafoveal telangiectasis. A fibrovascular mass and anastomoses are visible in the right eye.

f Color photograph in the same patient with stage 5 bilateral idiopathic juxtafoveal telangiectasis. A fibrovascular mass and a yellowish milky reflex temporal to the fovea are seen in the left eye.

g Arteriovenous phase in the left eye. Capillary ectasias and staining of a choroidal neovascularization are seen.

h Late arteriovenous phase in the left eye. There is leakage from the affected capillaries and from the choroidal neovascular vessels.

i Late phase. There is a slight increase in the leakage. There was no evidence of edema either on ophthalmoscopy or optical coherence tomography; the patient's visual acuity was 1.0.

7.11 Radiation Retinopathy   *Lothar Krause*

Epidemiology, Pathophysiology, and Clinical Presentation

- Radiation retinopathy is a retinal vessel disease caused by the damaging effects of protons, beta rays, or gamma rays on the structure of vessel walls.
- This type of retinopathy can develop after external beam radiotherapy, after brachytherapy with ruthenium or iodine plaques, or after proton beam radiation. The severity depends on the dosage (starting at about 30 Gy), the size of the irradiated surface, and the type of fractionation used. Radiation retinopathy is observed more frequently in diabetic patients.
- Radiation retinopathy typically appears several months or years after the radiotherapy, due to chronic vessel wall damage. Clinically, occlusive vasculopathy becomes visible in the form capillary occlusions and ischemic areas with microaneurysms, retinal hemorrhage, retinal edema, macular edema, and exudates. Neovascularizations may also develop (on the optic disc, retina, or iris).
- Radiation retinopathy is not limited to the areas that receive the maximum radiation energy, but can also be detected in vessels lying outside of the center of the radiation field.
- When the optic nerve head is involved, swelling of the optic nerve head and parapapillary hemorrhage (radiation neuropathy) may be observed, with progression to atrophy optic nerve.

Fluorescein Angiography

- The clinical picture is characteristic and is usually sufficient for diagnosis in patients with a history of radiation exposure. Fluorescein angiography makes it possible to identify avascular areas and also facilitates laser photocoagulation.
- Areas of hyperfluorescence appear on the optic nerve head in the early phase, as a result of leakage. Hypo-

fluorescence can be seen as a result of capillary occlusions and hemorrhage or retinal edema (or exudates).
- The arteriovenous phase shows areas of hyperfluorescence along the vessels, resulting from increased permeability of the damaged vessel walls, and dot-shaped areas of hyperfluorescence caused by microaneurysms and telangiectases.
- There is an increase in the areas of hyperfluorescence in the late phase, and cystoid macular edema can also be found in some cases.

Diagnosis and Treatment

- The case history and the clinical picture determine the diagnosis. Fluorescein angiography can confirm the location of the ischemic areas, capillary occlusions, microaneurysms, proliferations, and macular edema.
- The treatment depends on the degree and location of the vessel damage. As in other occlusive retinal diseases, panretinal laser coagulation is used to prevent or treat neovascularization. The prognosis for the preservation of visual acuity is very limited with radiation neuropathy, although cases of spontaneous resolution have been reported.

References

Brown GC, Shields JA, Sanborn G, Augsburger JJ, Savino PJ, Schatz NJ. Radiation retinopathy. Ophthalmology 1982;89:1494–501.

Gunduz K, Shields CL, Shields JA, Cater J, Freire JE, Brady LW. Radiation retinopathy following plaque radiotherapy for posterior uveal melanoma. Arch Ophthalmol 1999;117:609–14.

Spaide RF, Leys A, Herrmann-Delemazure B, et al. Radiation-associated choroidal neovasculopathy. Ophthalmology 1999;106:2254–60.

Takahashi K, Kishi S, Muraoka K, Tanaka T, Shimizu K. Radiation choroidopathy with remodeling of the choroidal venous system. Am J Ophthalmol 1998;125:367–73.

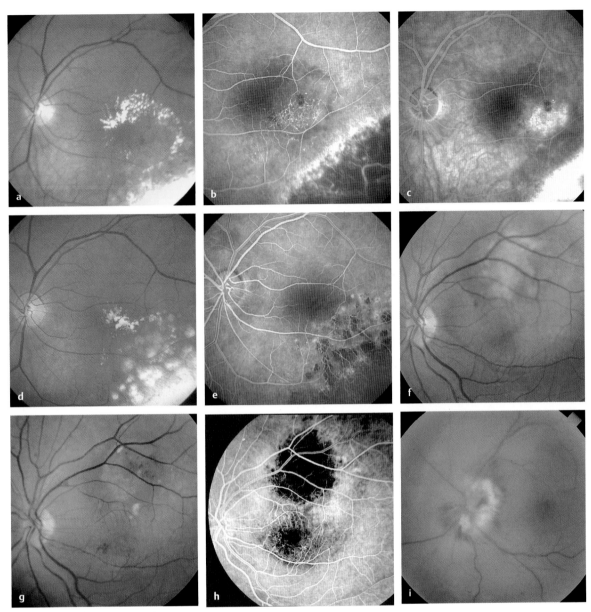

Fig. 7.11a–i Radiation retinopathy

a Color photograph. The edge of a radiation scar after ruthenium plaque radiotherapy for a choroidal melanoma can be seen in the lower part of the image. Beyond the radiation scar, microaneurysms, dot hemorrhages, hard exudates, and macular edema are all visible at the posterior pole.

b Arteriovenous phase. Central to the scar, an area with telangiectatic neovascularization, small, dot-like extravascular areas of hyperfluorescence in the microaneurysms, and leakage are visible as signs of vessel wall damage. The clinically visible hard exudates are no longer identifiable. The choroidal vessels are visible in the radiation scar as a result of damage to the retinal pigment epithelium and choriocapillaris.

c Late phase. There is increasing leakage in the area described above, up to and into the fovea, with reduced visual acuity. Hyperfluorescence is also visible in the area of the radiation scar.

d Color photograph. The same patient, with regression of the central exudates visible 6 months after laser coagulation of the affected area.

e Arteriovenous phase. Markedly fewer telangiectatic vessels are visible. The choroidal vessels are recognizable in the areas of laser treatment and radiation scarring.

f Color photograph. A choroidal melanoma with orange pigment in the upper temporal vessel arcade.

g Color photograph. Cotton-wool spots and hemorrhages indicating vessel damage and radiation retinopathy at the posterior pole are recognizable after proton therapy.

h Arteriovenous phase. There are areas of hypofluorescence due to blockage in the tumor area. Telangiectatic vessel alterations in the parafoveal capillary network are recognizable outside of the actual radiation field in the macula. These subsequently lead to further leakage and thus to macular edema.

i Color photograph. Radiation neuropathy in a different patient after proton-beam therapy for a large choroidal melanoma in the nasal area (tumor not shown).

8.1 Central Serous Chorioretinopathy   *Werner Inhoffen*

Epidemiology, Pathophysiology, and Clinical Presentation

- Central serous chorioretinopathy can be described as neurosensory detachment resulting from idiopathic pigment epithelial leakage and can be divided into two basic types:
  - Classic central serous chorioretinopathy, with one or more areas of focal leakage.
  - Diffuse pigment epitheliopathy (chronic central serous chorioretinopathy; see section 8.2).
- The term most often used for this disease in the German-language literature is "retinitis centralis serosa," which dates back to the era of Albrecht von Graefe. The disease is more commonly known as "idiopathic central serous chorioretinopathy" (ICSC). The term "central serous retinopathy" (CSR) is also often used.
- In most cases, the etiology remains unclear; these cases are therefore classified as idiopathic central serous chorioretinopathy. Pathogenetically, a localized permeability dysfunction of the choroid is suspected. Secondary central serous chorioretinopathy can be observed during pregnancy, in patients receiving systemic steroids (including occasional inhalation), after organ transplantation, and in patients with glomerulonephritis, Crohn disease, or choroidal folds.
- The disease predominantly affects patients between the ages of 20 and 50, and mainly presents unilaterally. The proportion of men to women is 2.7 : 1; 60–90 % present with acute central serous chorioretinopathy and 5–40 % present with chronic central serous retinopathy.
- The most common symptoms of the disease are a deterioration in visual acuity, micropsia, metamorphopsia, reduced dark adaptation, color vision deficiencies, and a brownish spot in the central field of vision.
- Clinically, neurosensory detachments in the foveal area without pigment epithelial detachments can be observed, with multiple leakages in up to 30 % of patients. Patients with central pigment epithelial detachment are rare, and those with a bullous form are very rare.
- Recurrences may develop in about 30 % of patients during the course of the disease, and can even occur three or more times in approximately 10 % of patients.

Fluorescein and Indocyanine Green Angiography

- An umbrella or "smokestack" pattern can be seen in approximately a quarter of the cases, starting with a small hyperfluorescent spot in the arteriovenous phase, with leakage that continues upward in the course of the angiography and then spreads downward along the neurosensory detachment borders.
- In approximately 60 % of cases, what is known as an "expanding pinpoint" can be identified as a hyperfluorescent spot in the early phase, which enlarges in all directions simultaneously afterward.
- A spot with a minimally increasing hyperfluorescent area can be found in approximately 15 % of cases.

- One spot is seen in most cases, but two or more hyperfluorescent spots with leakage can be found in up to approximately 30 %.
- Indocyanine green angiography reveals hyperfluorescent, expanding areas, which are also usually visible in the unaffected areas and can often be detected in the fellow eye.

Diagnosis and Treatment

- The diagnosis is based on typical symptoms and ophthalmoscopy, which reveals a nearly round central neurosensory detachment with transparent serous subretinal fluid and no evidence of choroidal neovascularization. The diagnosis is established by fluorescein angiography.
- The prognosis is generally good, especially if the initial visual acuity is 0.5 or better (95 % of patients achieve visual acuity of more than 0.63). The recovery period averages approximately 4 months. Healing usually leads to defects in the retinal pigment epithelium and can leave persistent metamorphopsia.
- Important, and occasionally difficult, differential diagnoses are: idiopathic choroidal neovascularization, neurosensory detachment associated with optic pit, polypoidal choroidal vasculopathy, and retinal telangiectasia. With stereo angiography, telangiectases only show leakages in the retinal layers.
- The most widely advocated treatment method at present is localized laser coagulation of the original pigment epithelial defect. There have as yet been no controlled prospective studies.
- The majority of published papers state that laser coagulation reduces the duration of the illness, but it does not improve the final visual acuity in comparison with untreated eyes. The complication rate (with the development of choroidal neovascularization resulting from laser treatment) is 1–5 %. As spontaneous resolution takes 3–5 months on average, most authors only recommend laser photocoagulation for patients with persistent leakage and symptoms that have persisted for 6 months or longer.
- Some authors state that systemic acetazolamide therapy can shorten the recovery period in acute central serous retinopathy, but this treatment apparently has no influence on the final visual acuity.
- Systemic corticosteroid therapy is contraindicated.

References

Piccolino FC, Borgia L, Zinicola E, Zingirian M. Indocyanine green angiographic findings in central serous chorioretinopathy. Eye 1995; 9:324–32.

Robertson DM. Argon laser photocoagulation treatment in central serous chorioretinopathy. Ophthalmology 1986;93:972–4.

Yamada K, Hayasaka S, Setogawa T. Fluorescein-angiographic patterns in patients with central serous chorioretinopathy at the initial visit. Ophthalmologica 1992;205:69–76.

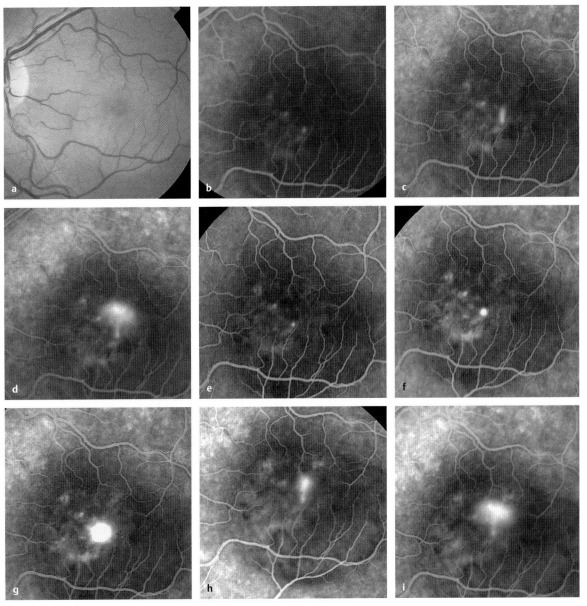

Fig. 8.**1a–i Central serous chorioretinopathy**

a Color photograph. Acute central serous chorioretinopathy, with a slightly yellow central neurosensory detachment.

b Early arteriovenous phase. Blocked fluorescence caused by the exudate inside the detachment; an irregular hyperfluorescent surface with three hyperfluorescent points can be seen inside.

c Late arteriovenous phase. One of these leaking points expands upward, creating a smokestack appearance.

d Late phase. The leakage continues expanding upward and starts to occupy the hollow space in the neurosensory detachment.

e Early arteriovenous phase. The same patient, 3 months later. No significant difference is recognizable in the early arteriovenous phase in comparison with the initial examination.

f Late arteriovenous phase. The smokestack is no longer visible, but there is a flat expansion of the hyperfluorescence from the source point (the "expanding pinpoint" appearance).

g Late phase. Further radial expansion of the hyperfluorescence, but no umbrella pattern.

h Late arteriovenous phase. The same patient, another 3 months later. No significant differences from the angiography carried out at the first visit are evident.

i Late phase. The same smokestack appearance as at the first visit, with increasing neurosensory detachment. This patient therefore has different angiographic signs during acute central serous chorioretinopathy.

8.2 Chronic Central Serous Chorioretinopathy   *Werner Inhoffen*

Epidemiology, Pathophysiology, and Clinical Presentation

- In the English-language literature, chronic central serous chorioretinopathy is also known as diffuse retinal pigment epitheliopathy after its most obvious characteristic. Typically, diffuse areas of atrophy of the retinal pigment epithelium can be seen, with flat neurosensory detachments and pigment epithelial detachments. The course of the disease is chronic, and regular deterioration is common.
- Overall, the clinical picture is similar to that in acute central serous retinopathy, but the patients are mostly older (over 50), have distinct areas of atrophy of the retinal pigment epithelium with visual field defects (70%), and often suffer bilateral involvement (90%). In comparison with acute central serous chorioretinopathy, choroidal neovascularizations (CNV) develop in a larger proportion of the patients.
- The disease can either develop independently, or from recurrences of acute central serous chorioretinopathy.
- Retinal edema can sometimes be detected in the affected areas.

Fluorescein Angiography

- Small pinpoint-like leakages within a pigment epithelial atrophy are typical; they are frequently in a peripapillary location, are chronic and recurrent, and lack the strong leakage that can be seen in leakage areas associated with acute central serous retinopathy.
- Nonleaking defects in the retinal pigment epithelium almost always form in the area of earlier detachment of the neurosensory retina.

Indocyanine Green Angiography

- Indocyanine green angiography shows areas of diffuse leakage, with dispersion during the 30-minute late phase, which are similar to those in central serous chorioretinopathy but considerably more pronounced.

Diagnosis and Treatment

- A long-term disease course, with phases of clinical improvement and deterioration, is typical.
- The differential diagnosis from occult CNV in age-related macular degeneration is often difficult. Follow-up is therefore necessary before the diagnosis is conclusively established, with the help of indocyanine green angiography if necessary. Hemorrhages—a classic aspect of CNVs—expansion of the lesion, and retinal edema, argue against the existence of chronic central serous retinopathy alone.
- To prevent further secondary damage as a result of detachment (visual field defects, damage or atrophy of the retinal pigment epithelium, loss of vision), some authors recommend grid laser coagulation in the area of diffuse leakage.

References

Cohen D, Gaudric A, Coscas G, Quentel G, Binaghi M. [Diffuse retinal epitheliopathy and central serous chorioretinopathy; in French.] J Fr Ophtalmol 1983;6:339–49.

Iide T, Yannuzzi LA, Spaide RF, et al. Chronic central serous chorioretinopathy. Retina 2003;23:1–7.

Lafaut BA, Salati C, Priem H, De Laey JJ. Indocyanine green angiography is of value for the diagnosis of chronic central serous chorioretinopathy in elderly patients. Graefes Arch Clin Exp Ophthalmol 1998;236:513–21.

Levine R, Brucker AJ, Robinson F. Long-term follow-up of idiopathic central serous chorioretinopathy by fluorescein angiography. Ophthalmology 1989;96:854–9.

Spaide RF, Campeas L, Haas A, et al. Central serous chorioretinopathy in younger and older adults. Ophthalmology 1996;103:2070–80.

Yannuzzi LA, Slakter JS, Kaufman SR, Gupta K. Laser treatment of diffuse retinal pigment epitheliopathy. Eur J Ophthalmol 1992;2:103–14.

8

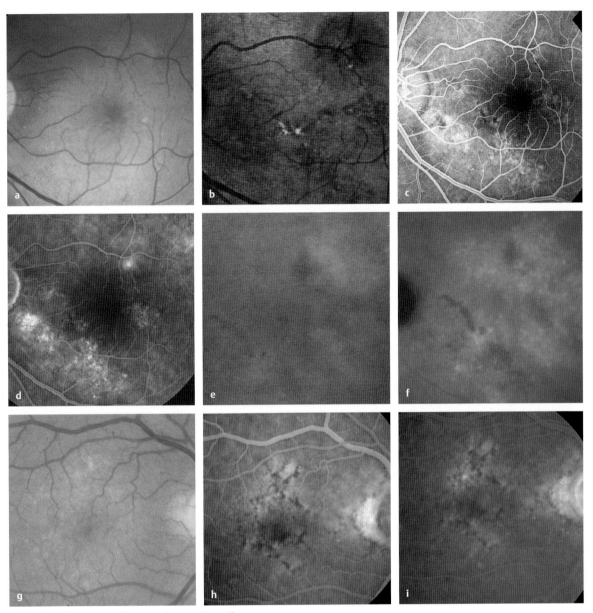

Fig. 8.**2a–i Chronic central serous chorioretinopathy**

a Color photograph. Chronic and acute central serous chorioretinopathy, with no foveal reflex and detachment of the neurosensory retina extrafoveal at the 2-o'clock position.

b Infrared image. Confocal infrared ophthalmoscopy with the scanning laser ophthalmoscope accentuates a flat detachment of the
neurosensory retina along the temporal lower vessel arcade, as
well as an acute detachment at the 2-o'clock position, shown as a
dark area.

c Arteriovenous phase. Detachment of the neurosensory retina at
the 2-o'clock position and defects in the retinal pigment
epithelium along the temporal lower vessel arcade.

d Late phase. There is a point with strong leakage at the 2-o'clock
position (acute central serous chorioretinopathy) and diffuse,
moderate leakage in the area with retinal pigment epithelium defects at the temporal lower vessel arcade (chronic central serous
chorioretinopathy).

e Indocyanine green angiography, at 10 min. Hyperfluorescence
and initial leakage in the area of the acute and chronic central serous chorioretinopathy can be seen.

f Indocyanine green angiography, at 30 min. There is expansion of
the Indocyanine green central hyperfluorescence as well as at the
2-o'clock position.

g Color photograph in a patient with an occult choroidal neovascularization. A mixed image of atrophies and pigment clumping can
be seen. Retinal edema can be confirmed using optical coherence
tomography.

h Arteriovenous phase. Hypofluorescent and hyperfluorescent
areas that match the fundus findings.

i Late phase. There is mild diffuse and localized leakage in the temporal area above the fovea.

8.3 Macular Pucker   *Werner Inhoffen*

Epidemiology, Pathophysiology, and Clinical Presentation

- The epiretinal development of gliosis in the macula, with distortion of the retina and resulting dysfunction, is known as idiopathic epiretinal gliosis (when a peripheral retina hole is not detectable) or macular pucker (when gliosis is secondary to formation of a retinal break or retinal detachment). The distinction between these two groups is vague, since in idiopathic epiretinal gliosis, small peripheral holes (which are clinically not always diagnosable) can often be found in postmortem examinations.
- In addition to the idiopathic group and classic macular pucker, epimacular membranes can also develop after other vitreoretinal diseases or therapy (branch retinal vein occlusion, uveitis, laser coagulation, and ocular tumor therapy).
- In practice, the term "macular pucker" has emerged as the generic term for these three types of epiretinal gliosis.
- Histologically, the membranes consist of collagens, partly from internal limiting membranes, retinal pigment epithelial cells, astrocytes, fibrocytes, and macrophages.
- The retinal vessels can become irregularly distorted by the epiretinal membrane resulting in edema. The membrane can overgrow the fovea, resulting in increased macular thickness without cysts and without foveal depression, or can create a macular full-thickness hole by tangential traction of the epiretinal membrane.
- The prevalence is 6% in patients over the age of 50; the disease is bilateral in 20–30% of cases.
- The patient usually notices a decrease in visual acuity with metamorphopsia within a few weeks, followed by a period of relative stability or only a slow deterioration in visual acuity. Only about 1% of patients with macular pucker experience spontaneous separation of the membrane from the macula. Visual acuity deteriorates rapidly if a macular hole develops as a result of the pucker.

Fluorescein Angiography

- On angiography, the typical, sometimes corkscrew-shaped vessels are easier to identify as a result of improved contrast. In most cases, only moderately diffuse leakages can be detected in areas of disturbed vessels without the development of retinal cysts.
- Slight blurring above the distorted vessels may also result from thick epiretinal membranes.
- The diagnosis of a macular pucker is usually based on the clinical findings, without the assistance of angiography. However, in case of doubt, angiography is helpful for determining and identifying other causes (choroidal neovascularizations, telangiectasia, branch retinal vein occlusion).
- The extent of the leakage visible on angiography has no prognostic significance in relation to the expected postoperative results.

Diagnosis and Treatment

- The flat, glistening reflection of the gliosis is usually visible on ophthalmoscopy, particularly with the red-free light on the slitlamp. Additional signs include distortions of the vessels, puckering of the internal limiting membrane and absence of the fovea reflex, pseudoholes, or the development of a macular hole resulting from the puckering.
- Pars plana vitrectomy with membrane peeling is the standard treatment for symptomatic macular pucker, and leads to a comprehensive decrease in retinal thickness and consequent improvement in vision in more than 50% of cases. Full visual acuity cannot always be retained after this surgical procedure, since in many cases the foveal thickness does not return to normal values, particularly after a long-standing epimacular membrane.
- The value of additional peeling of internal limiting membranes and the application of dyes (indocyanine green or trypan blue) for intraoperative membrane staining has not been yet been clearly defined by prospective studies.

References

Charles S. Epimacular membranes. In: Guyer DR, Yannuzzi L, Chang S, eds. Retina–vitreous–macula. London: Saunders, 1999: 230–7.

Maguire AM, Margherio RR, Dmuchowski C. Preoperative fluorescein angiographic features of surgically removed idiopathic epiretinal membranes. Retina 1994;14:411–6.

Massin P, Allouch C, Haouchine B, et al. Optical coherence tomography of idiopathic macular epiretinal membranes before and after surgery. Am J Ophthalmol 2000;130:732–9.

Park DW, Dugel PU, Garda J, et al. Macular pucker removal with and without internal limiting membrane peeling: pilot study. Ophthalmology 2003;110:62–4.

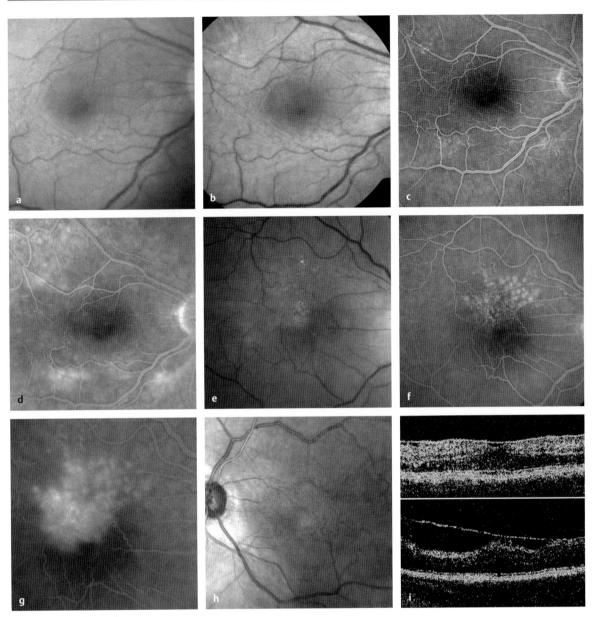

Fig. 8.3a–i Macular pucker

a Color photograph. Epiretinal gliosis; the foveal reflex is absent.

b Red-free imaging. Improved visualization of the epiretinal gliosis.

c Late arteriovenous phase. Distorted retinal vessels, with only moderate leakage.

d Late phase. The leakage has increased.

e A patient with focal laser coagulation after branch retinal vein occlusion who subsequently developed epiretinal gliosis, clearly visible with red-free imaging.

f Arteriovenous phase. Collateral vessels, laser scars, and a region with an occluded vessel are clearly visible.

g Late phase. The leakage is well demarcated, strong, and homogeneous, and is located in the region of distorted vessels—in contrast to leakage due to an epiretinal membrane.

h Infrared image. Macular pucker at the posterior pole with multiple wrinkles on the retina.

i Optical coherence tomography (different patient). In the upper image, epiretinal membrane formation and traction on the fovea is detectable. In some cases, traction is also present more peripherally (lower image).

8.4 Macular Holes   *Werner Inhoffen*

Epidemiology, Pathophysiology, and Clinical Presentation

- Impairment of foveal anatomy can be caused by tangential forces (in epiretinal gliosis) or by anterior–posterior traction (in vitreomacular traction syndrome). In both cases, the clinical presentation may range from a foveal defect with the formation of lamellar macular hole to a full-thickness macular hole.
- In the Gass classification, macular holes are divided into stages 1–4. Stage 1a is simply the absence of foveal depression; stage 1b is small areas with a full-thickness hole; and stages 2–4 is full-thickness holes. Further distinctions can be made depending on the diameter of the hole (400 µm: stages 2–3) and whether or not there is complete posterior vitreous detachment (stages 3–4). In the future, optical coherence tomography will probably lead to an improved classification.
- Lesions known as pseudoholes (the appearance of a hole due to a central break in an epiretinal membrane) and lamellar macular holes (in which a substantial part of the intact retinal tissue still remains central—e. g., after the collapse of a foveal cyst) have to be distinguished from full-thickness macular holes. One-third of all pseudoholes progress to full-thickness holes within 3 years.
- The prevalence of idiopathic macular holes in the USA amounts to approximately one in every 5000 patients. The majority of macular holes are idiopathic and unilateral at the beginning of the disease, and only a few arise as a result of trauma. Secondary holes due to other diseases have to be differentiated from idiopathic macular holes (e. g., after cystoid macular edema, in epiretinal membranes, in vitreoretinal traction syndrome, or in high myopia with staphyloma).
- Subjective symptoms initially include metamorphopsia and blurring of vision. In small vertical tractions, individual areas of printed text cannot be seen during reading. The development of a hole results in excentric fixation dystopia and thus leads to a drastic decline in visual acuity. Spontaneous occlusion of the hole is possible in stages 1 and 2; very often however, the findings deteriorate in all stages: 50 % in stages 1–2, 70 % in stages 2–3.
- When a macular hole appears in one eye, the risk of a hole developing in the fellow eye is approximately 10 % within 5–36 months after the first diagnosis. An important risk factor is an incomplete posterior vitreous detachment in the fellow eye.

Fluorescein Angiography

- Fluorescein angiography only has a minor role in the diagnosis of macular holes, in comparison with stereoscopic fundus examination and optical coherence tomography.

- It is not possible to distinguish between macular holes, pseudoholes, and lamellar holes to any degree of certainty using angiography. However, a stage 2–4 macular hole should be suspected if, after angiography, central, clearly defined, single window defects without leakage appear as a result of macular pigment displacement. The central window defect may disappear after successful closure of the hole.
- Angiography is clinically relevant for the differential diagnosis from cystoid macular edema, as these two entities cannot always be differentiated from each other clinically with any degree of certainty.

Diagnosis and Treatment

- Ophthalmoscopically, stage 3 and 4 holes are the easiest to recognize as darker central circular areas surrounded by a ring of elevated retina, sometimes also with small yellow deposits.
- In stage 1a, only a loss of the foveal reflex can be seen, sometimes combined with a light yellow spot. In stage 1b, the macular retinal pigment is pushed aside slightly, resulting in a fine yellow ring instead of a central yellow spot. The Watzke test (in which a narrow beam is projected onto the hole from the slit lamp) shows whether there is a central defect in the visual field; however, it is inaccurate for small holes. The findings of optical coherence tomography are particularly helpful, as they show the precise anatomical situation; the ophthalmoscopic classification alone is not always accurate.
- Vitrectomy, as a surgical treatment option, generally leads to good anatomic and functional results. The surgical technique is still variable at present (with alternatives including the administration of indocyanine green or trypan blue as vital stains for the removal of the internal limiting membrane, and different types of tamponade).

References

Chew EY, Sperduto RD, Hiller R, et al. Clinical course of macular holes: the Eye Disease Case–Control Study. Arch Ophthalmol 1999;117:242–6.

Gass JD. Reappraisal of biomicroscopic classification of stages of development of a macular hole. Am J Ophthalmol 1995;119:752–9.

La Cour M, Friis J. Macular holes: classification, epidemiology, natural history and treatment. Acta Ophthalmol Scand 2002;80:579–87.

Varano M, Scassa C, Capaldo N, Sciamanna M, Parisi V. Development of macular pseudoholes: a 36-month period of follow-up. Retina 2002;22:435–42.

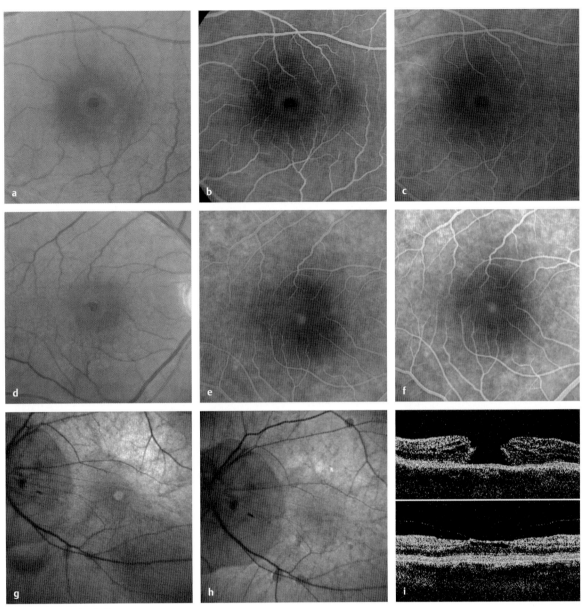

Fig. 8.**4a–i Macular holes**

a Color photograph. Stage 3 macular hole. There is a central defect with yellowish deposits. The edge of the hole is raised.

b Early arteriovenous phase. Only a small hyperfluorescent area is visible at the center of the defect. The raised edge is hyperfluorescent.

c Late phase. There is still no change and thus no leakage, in contrast to the findings in cystoid macular edema or choroidal neovascularization.

d Color photograph. Another patient with a similar clinical picture.

e The angiographic examination shows findings with differences from the previous patient. Even in the arteriovenous phase, the lesion is seen to have a central hyperfluorescent area, and the elevated retina is still hypofluorescent at the rim.

f Late phase. The findings are unchanged, with no significant leakage.

g Fundus autofluorescence (different patient): In this highly myopic patient the macular hole was difficult to detect clinically. Fundus autofluorescence is increased in the area of the hole due to absence of the overlying retina.

h Fundus autofluorescence (same patient as **g**). Six weeks after surgical closure of the hole fundus autofluorescence is normal in the fovea.

i Optical coherence tomography (different patient). Both eyes of one patient. The right eye (upper image) has a full-thickness macular hole. OCT imaging is even more useful to detect the impeding macular hole on the left eye (lower image).

8.5 Cystoid Macular Edema   *Werner Inhoffen*

Epidemiology, Pathophysiology, and Clinical Presentation

- Cystoid macular edema (CME) is an accumulation of fluid that leads to newly formed hollow spaces in the retina after various types of vitreoretinal disease.
- In diseases of the choroid, transfer of fluid from the choroid to the retina develops due to altered and permeable retinal pigment epithelium—e. g., in uveitis, multifocal choroiditis, choroidal (occult and classic) neovascularizations, and choroidal tumors.
- Increased permeability of the retinal vessels can be seen in diseases of the retina—e. g., in diabetic retinopathy, branch retinal vein occlusion, telangiectasia, radiation retinopathy, uveitis with involvement of retinal vessels (e. g., Behçet disease), Irvine–Gass syndrome, after yttrium–aluminum garnet (YAG) laser capsulotomy, epiretinal gliosis, laser coagulation, retinitis pigmentosa, and after filtering glaucoma surgery or vitreoretinal surgery.
- The fluid accumulates in hollow spaces between the external plexiform layer and the internal cell layer. Strictly speaking, these newly formed hollow spaces do not represent cysts because of the lack of epithelial lining. However, they can be classified as pseudocysts.
- The fovea is predominantly affected. Because of its specific anatomy (e. g., with a lack of stabilizing Müller cells), cysts can considerably increase in size in the area of the fovea.
- The clinical appearance is therefore typical, with only a few large central cysts surrounded by a ring of smaller cysts that decrease in size toward the periphery.
- Subjective symptoms in cystoid macular edema are generally metamorphopsia and a decrease in visual acuity.

Fluorescein Angiography

- Typically, angiography shows a slow accumulation of fluorescein in the cystoid spaces. These are centrally located with some large hyperfluorescences, mostly with fine hypofluorescent pigment rings; often, many small, almost round areas of hyperfluorescence can be seen toward the periphery in the later phases. A classification of the severity of cystoid macular edema (which is important in clinical studies) is available, but is not particularly useful in everyday practice.
- The typical angiographic picture of cystoid macular edema cannot be seen in macular holes, macular dystrophy, or solar retinopathy.

Diagnosis and Treatment

- The diagnosis is established on the basis of the case history, an evaluation of the underlying disease, and ophthalmoscopy.
- In slitlamp microscopy, the cysts are best demonstrated with a laterally orientated slit beam, as the scattered light reveals density changes inside the retina. Optical coherence tomography or angiography can be carried out to obtain supplementary information.
- Treatment is directed toward the underlying disease. Improvements have been achieved with systemic acetazolamide treatment, nonsteroidal anti-inflammatory therapy, and intravitreal or systemic corticosteroid administration.
- In persistent cystoid macular edema, there is a risk of a tear developing in the "roof" of a cyst, resulting in a lamellar macular hole. Vitrectomy with membrane peeling or perifoveal laser coagulation may be helpful in these cases before a hole develops.

References

Fishman GA, Gilbert LD, Fiscella RG, Kimura AE, Jampol LM. Acetazolamide for treatment of chronic macular edema in retinitis pigmentosa. Arch Ophthalmol 1989;107:1445–52.

Fu A, Ahmed I, Ai E. Cystoid macular edema. In: Yanoff M, Duker JS, eds. Ophthalmology. London: Mosby, 2nd ed., 2004:956–62.

Jonas JB, Kreissig I, Sofker A, Degenring RF. Intravitreal injection of triamcinolone for diffuse diabetic macular edema. Arch Ophthalmol 2003;121:57–61.

Otani T, Kishi S. A controlled study of vitrectomy for diabetic macular edema. Am J Ophthalmol 2002;134:214–9.

Ting TD, Oh M, Cox TA, Meyer CH, Toth CA. Decreased visual acuity associated with cystoid macular edema in neovascular age-related macular degeneration. Arch Ophthalmol 2002;120:731–7.

8

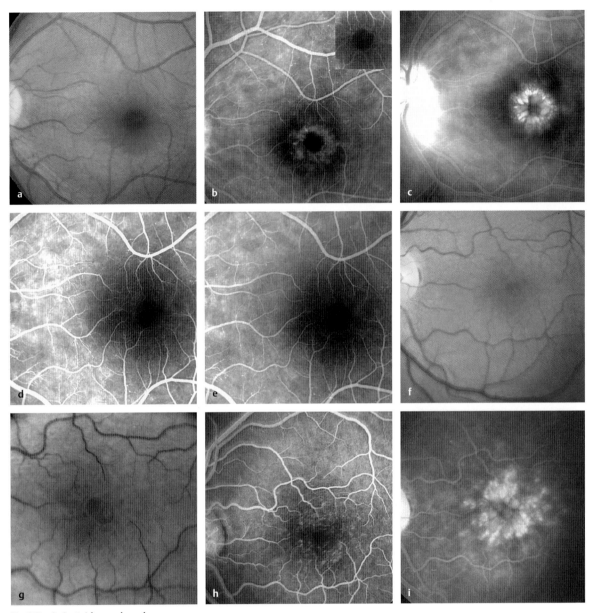

Fig. 8.**5a–i Cystoid macular edema**

a Color photograph. There is an absence of the foveal reflex in a patient with posterior uveitis.

b Early arteriovenous phase (inset): the perifoveal capillaries appear virtually normal, but small hyperfluorescences can be seen at the 11-o'clock position. Late arteriovenous phase (large image): leakage from the perifoveal capillaries and formation of radially orientated areas of leakage can be seen.

c Late phase. There is an accumulation of dye in the hollow spaces formed by the edema. The largest "cysts" are located in the center, and they decrease in size toward the periphery.

d Same patient one month after interferone alpha-2a therapy: Late arteriovenous phase. No leakage can be seen after regression of the cystoid macular edema.

e Late phase. There is almost no leakage, and there is no cystoid pattern.

f Color photograph. Clearly visible central cysts in a female patient after implantation of an intraocular lens (Irvine–Gass syndrome).

g Red-free image. The extent of the cystoid macular edema is easier to document using a red-free 20° digital exposure, as the small cysts can also be demonstrated with high contrast using this technique.

h Early arteriovenous phase. Dye is starting to be released from the perifoveal capillaries.

i Late phase. There is an accumulation of dye in the preformed hollow spaces, with the typical pattern of cystoid macular edema.

8

8.6 Choroidal Folds, Choroidal Ruptures, and Angioid Streaks   *Werner Inhoffen*

Choroidal Folds

- Choroidal folds are parallel continuous creases of choroid and retinal pigment epithelium in the area of the posterior pole. Depending on the cause, these can be unilateral or bilateral, and they can present in combination with the following changes:
  - Idiopathic choroidal folds in hyperopic patients, often bilateral, occasionally with minor impairment of vision.
  - In ocular hypotony, due to reduced intraocular pressure (e. g., after filtering glaucoma surgery).
  - In uveitis—e. g., in chronic optic disc swelling and posterior scleritis.
  - In retrobulbar space-occupying lesions (endocrine orbitopathy, tumors, mucocele) causing indentation of the eye due to space constriction.
  - In scar formation in the choroidal or in the subretinal space—e. g., in the fibrotic stage of an advanced age-related macular degeneration.
  - In space-occupying lesions in the choroid (e. g., malignant choroidal melanoma).
- Subjectively, the choroidal folds can remain asymptomatic, or can lead to metamorphopsia and a reduction in visual acuity.
- Because of their wave-like arrangement and the resulting local changes in the density of the pigment epithelial cells, ophthalmoscopy shows parallel dark lines, which are mainly slanting or horizontal, but can also be occasionally vertical, combined with less pigmented lines in between. In the unilateral forms, scleritis, tumors, vessel occlusions, and hypotony are the most common causes (each approximately 13–17%), followed by age-related macular degeneration (10%), whereas in the bilateral form, age-related macular degeneration, hypotony, and idiopathic forms together amount to 75%.

Fluorescein Angiography

- Typical hypofluorescent and slightly hyperfluorescent lines can be seen, running in parallel and without leakage, as well as only hyperfluorescent lines occasionally. The pattern depends on the configuration of the folds. The hypofluorescence is caused by increased pigmentation due to compression of the retinal pigment epithelium at the bottom of the folds; the hyperfluorescence is due to decreased pigmentation resulting from thinning of the retinal pigment epithelium on top of the folds.
- The areas of hyperfluorescence increase during the course of the angiography procedure; however, leakage is not found.

Diagnosis and Treatment

- Choroidal folds are easily recognizable on ophthalmoscopy, but are easier to identify with fluorescein angiography. This disease pattern has to be differentiated from retinal folds (e. g., there is no evidence of gliosis) and pure retinal pigment epithelium folds in age-related macular degeneration.
- The treatment is based on the initial cause of the choroidal folds.

References

Cassidy LM, Sanders MD. Choroidal folds and papilloedema. Br J Ophthalmol 1999;83:1139–43.

Leahey AB, Brucker AJ, Wyszynski RE, Shaman P. Chorioretinal folds: a comparison of unilateral and bilateral cases. Arch Ophthalmol 1993;111:357–9.

Von Winning CH. Fluography of choroidal folds. Doc Ophthalmol 1972;31:209–49.

Choroidal Ruptures _____

Epidemiology, Pathophysiology, and Clinical Presentation

- The following anatomical changes can occur in the retinal and choroidal areas following blunt trauma:
  - Berlin edema, with subsequent pigment displacement and reduction in visual acuity, depending on the location.
  - Macular holes/retinal breaks.
  - Choroidal rupture.
- Multiple choroidal ruptures can often be found at the posterior pole. On ophthalmoscopy, these can be identified as arched, light streaks with pigment displacements, orientated around the optic nerve. They are often masked by subretinal hemorrhages, which are slowly absorbed, resulting in increased visual acuity after absorption.
- A permanent reduction in visual acuity can result from secondary pigment changes (approximately 7% of cases).
- The frequency of secondary choroidal neovascularization lies between 14% and 20% and increases the nearer the rupture lies to the fovea and the larger it is. Choroidal neovascularization may develop within 6 weeks, but can also emerge from the scar years later.

Fluorescein Angiography

- Often, only parts of a rupture are visible due to masking hemorrhage. In addition to fluorescein angiography, indocyanine green angiography may therefore also be necessary to eliminate the possibility of a choroidal neovascularization.
- In the early phase of fluorescein angiography, hypofluorescence can be seen in the ruptured area, with later hyperfluorescence resulting from staining of the damaged tissue. The hemorrhages remain hypofluorescent.

Indocyanine Green Angiography

- The whole extent of the rupture can be detected in indocyanine green angiography, and choroidal neovascularization obscured by hemorrhage can be excluded or detected.
- Indocyanine green angiography often reveals more ruptures than can be seen with ophthalmoscopy or fluorescein angiography.

Diagnosis and Treatment

- The diagnosis is based on ophthalmoscopy and fluorescein angiography, both of which are recommended when choroidal neovascularization is suspected.
- Generally, treatment is only administered if complications arise—i.e., if a choroidal neovascularization develops. There have not as yet been any prospective and controlled studies. Choroidal neovascularizations can be treated using laser coagulation, photodynamic therapy, or surgery.

References

Giuffre G. [Traumatic choroid tears: visual prognosis and long-term course; in French.] J Fr Ophtalmol 1988;11:569–77.

Kohno T, Miki T, Shiraki K, Kano K, Hirabayashi-Matsushita M. Indocyanine green angiographic features of choroidal rupture and choroidal vascular injury after contusion ocular injury. Am J Ophthalmol 2000;129:38–46.

Secretan M, Sickenberg M, Zografos L, Piguet B. Morphometric characteristics of traumatic choroidal ruptures associated with neovascularization. Retina 1998;18:62–6.

8

Angioid Streaks _____

Epidemiology, Pathophysiology, and Clinical Presentation

- Angioid streaks are continuous defects at the posterior pole that continue into the Bruch membrane area and change the pigment epithelium, forming dark, broad, curved lines. The initial ophthalmoscopic findings create the impression of unusual additional vessels, particularly around the optic nerve head, where a peripapillary ring often forms. The "streaks" can intersect and often run through the fovea area without interfering with vision.
- Histologically, the Bruch membrane is often calcified, fragmented, and broken, and choroidal neovascularizations may consequently develop at this location. These are difficult to treat.
- Drusen of the optic nerve head, flat pigment displacement ("orange skin"), and peripheral "salmon spots" are also commonly encountered.
- In 50% of patients, angioid streaks are a sign of generalized disease:
  - Pseudoxanthoma elasticum (the most common)—some 85% of these patients develop eye abnormalities (Grönblad–Strandberg syndrome).
  - Ehlers–Danlos syndrome (rare).
- Subjectively, symptoms are only noted if impaired vision becomes evident due to choroidal neovascularization, usually with hemorrhage.

Fluorescein Angiography

- In early exposures, slightly hyperfluorescent, vessel-like streaks can be seen, but these are not associated with dye filling or leakage—with the exception of newly formed vessels (choroidal neovascularization).
- Early signs, with small, bright, almost round hyperfluorescent spots—sometimes with leakage, but not yet showing the vascular patterns that suggest choroidal neovascularization—are important for early recognition of choroidal neovascularizations in angioid streaks.

Indocyanine Green Angiography

- Indocyanine green angiography can be used for clear demonstration of further details—e.g., choroidal neovascularization covered with subretinal blood.

Diagnosis and Treatment

- The diagnosis can generally be made with ophthalmoscopy alone, but angiography reveals more angioid streaks and can detect choroidal neovascularizations.
- Choroidal ruptures, lacquer cracks in myopia. and pigment displacement in age-related macular degeneration all have to be differentiated diagnostically.
- There is no treatment for angioid streaks, but a medical and dermatological examination should also be carried out (due to possible vascular complications elsewhere).
- If choroidal neovascularization develops treatment similar to established regimens in age-related macular degeneration is suggested. In angioid streaks recurrences that develop frequently after only a short time limit a long-term success.
- Choroidal rupture may also occur after minor blunt trauma to the globe, because of the generally brittle tissue in the Bruch membrane area at the posterior pole.

References

Lim JI, Bressler NM, Marsh MJ, Bressler SB. Laser treatment of choroidal neovascularization in patients with angioid streaks. Am J Ophthalmol 1993;116:414–23.

Pece A, Avanza P, Introini U, Brancato R. Indocyanine green angiography in angioid streaks. Acta Ophthalmol Scand 1997;75:261–5.

Sato K, Ikeda T. Fluorescein angiographic features of neovascular maculopathy in angioid streaks. Jpn J Ophthalmol 1994;38:417–22.

Shaikh S, Ruby AJ, Williams GA. Photodynamic therapy using verteporfin for choroidal neovascularization in angioid streaks. Am J Ophthalmol 2003;135:1–6.

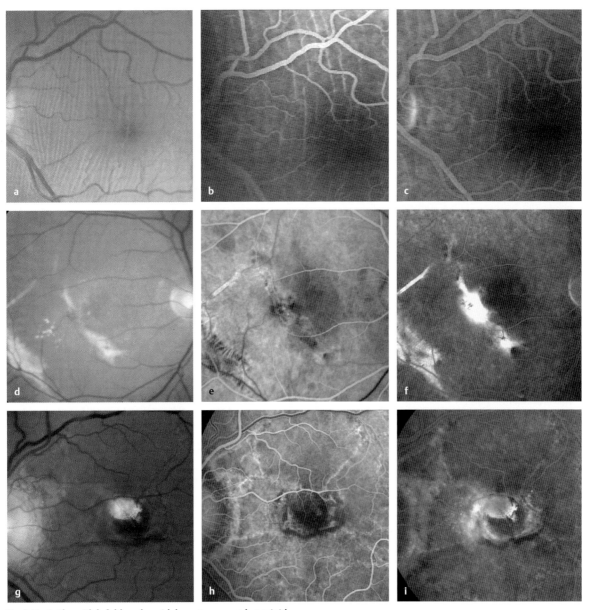

Fig. 8.6a–i Choroidal folds, choroidal ruptures, and angioid streaks

a Color photograph. Choroidal folds as a result of a mucocele nasal to the optic nerve head are seen. Dark and bright, parallel streaks are visible.

b Late arteriovenous phase. Bright parallel streaks are visible, corresponding to the choroidal folds.

c Late phase. The hyperfluorescent streaks are unchanged; no leakage is visible.

d Color photograph. An old choroidal rupture with choroidal neovascularization. There is a scarred choroidal rupture line temporal to the fovea, with reddish, slightly fibrosed irregularities.

e Early phase. The vessels in the choroidal neovascularization inside the central rupture are clearly visible. The rupture itself is hypofluorescent, with intersecting choroidal vessels.

f Late phase. Leakage from the choroidal neovascularization and staining of the fibrosed ruptures.

g Color photograph. Angioid streaks with a laser scar in secondary choroidal neovascularization and subsequent recurrence after treatment with photodynamic therapy. There is a dark angioid streak running through the fovea, above which a laser scar with central pigmentation can be seen. The laser scar has a fibrotic edge (recurrence).

h Early arteriovenous phase. Bright angioid streaks and a dark laser scar with surrounding choroidal neovascular vessels (recurrence) are visible.

i Late phase. There is no leakage from the streaks; staining of the laser scar fibrosis and the fibrotic recurrence is visible, but there is also leakage in the nasal, active part of a new classic and occult recurrence.

8

8.7 Light Injury to the Retina *Werner Inhoffen*

Epidemiology, Pathophysiology, and Clinical Presentation

- Solar retinopathy, iatrogenic phototoxicity due to the microscope or light-pipe, and accidental illumination of the eye by a laser beam can lead to acute light damage to the retina.
- Solar retinopathy. When the pupils are dilated and one gazes directly into the sun, the sun is projected onto the retina as a disc with a diameter of about 160 µm. The retina can warm up by an additional 22°, resulting in thermal damage. With a normal-sized pupil, a phototoxic reaction may be induced if the sun is viewed continuously for approximately 90 s (e.g., under the influence of drugs), resulting in a small limited edema directly in, or beside, the fovea. Direct observation of the sun through a telescope, with the resulting magnification, is extremely dangerous.
- A phototoxic reaction can also be produced on a larger surface area through iatrogenic phototoxicity caused by light from an operating microscope, or with light fibers used intraoperatively. These injuries are usually prevented nowadays through the use of special filters in the illumination path.
- Laser damage caused by industrial and military lasers mainly occurs due to Nd:YAG lasers in the infrared or visible spectrum. Direct coagulation is possible in these cases, as a higher focused energy can be applied to the eye. The lesions are similar to those caused by medical laser photocoagulation, but may be larger (e.g., similar to the size of a traumatic macular hole).
- Metamorphopsia and scotomas (causing reading difficulties) are often encountered in solar retinopathy or iatrogenic laser surgery, usually within 1 h, and are also often associated with a decrease in visual acuity. Hardly any symptoms accompany iatrogenic injury due to the operating microscope, as low-grade pigment changes can generally be seen outside of the visual center.
- Red laser pointers (available up to 5 mW) are considered harmless.

Fluorescein Angiography

- Leakages are not detectable in solar retinopathy. In some cases, a small window defect can develop if the lesion lies outside of the macular pigment blockage.
- A flat, moderate, extrafoveal window defect with indistinct borders develops in iatrogenic phototoxicity. Initial leakage is also visible in some cases.
- In laser accidents, the appearance depends on the energy and timing of application. Inconspicuous lesions, or lesions that are round or clearly defined, with leakage, blockage, and window defects can be found.

Diagnosis and Treatment

- The clinical findings in solar retinopathy consist of unilateral or bilateral large, round, yellow lesions, mainly 200 µm in size, close to the fovea. The healing process involves mild pigmentation. Small scotomas persist mainly as functional losses.
- In iatrogenic injury due to intraoperative light exposure, the damage depends on the location of the large, oval lesions, which usually range in size from half a disc diameter to two disc diameters (with a light yellow surface and some edema). Round lesions tend to occur when fiber optics have been used. The healing process involves pigment displacement, and the overall prognosis is good.
- In laser accidents, the prognosis depends on the location of the lesion and the extent of the injury.
- There is as yet no confirmed treatment for any of the three forms of light injury to the retina. Corticosteroid therapy, which is often administered, is still a matter of controversy. Particular attention should therefore be given to the preventing this type of injury, which is always avoidable.

References

Alhalel A, Glovinsky Y, Treister G, Bartov E, Blumenthal M, Belkin M. Long-term follow up of accidental parafoveal laser burns. Retina 1993;13:152–4.

Kleinmann G, Hoffman P, Schechtman E, Pollack A. Microscope-induced retinal phototoxicity in cataract surgery of short duration. Ophthalmology 2002;109:334–8.

MacFaul PA. Visual prognosis after solar retinopathy. Br J Ophthalmol 1969;53:534–41.

Michels M, Sternberg P Jr. Operating microscope-induced retinal phototoxicity: pathophysiology, clinical manifestations and prevention. Surv Ophthalmol 1990;34:237–52.

Michels M, Lewis H, Abrams GW, Han DP, Mieler WF, Neitz J. Macular phototoxicity caused by fiberoptic endoillumination during pars plana vitrectomy. Am J Ophthalmol 1992;114:287–96.

Pariselle J, Sastourne JC, Bidaux F, May F, Renard JP, Maurin JF. [Eye injuries caused by lasers in military and industrial environment. Apropos of 13 cases; in French.] J Fr Ophtalmol 1998;21:661–9.

Robertson DM, Lim TH, Salomao DR, Link TP, Rowe RL, McLaren JW. Laser pointers and the human eye: a clinicopathologic study. Arch Ophthalmol 2000;118:1686–91.

Thach AB, Lopez PF, Snady-McCoy LC, Golub BM, Frambach DA. Accidental Nd:YAG laser injuries to the macula. Am J Ophthalmol 1995;119:767–73.

Yannuzzi LA, Fisher YL, Krueger A, Slakter J. Solar retinopathy: a photobiological and geophysical analysis. Trans Am Ophthalmol Soc 1987;85:120–8.

8

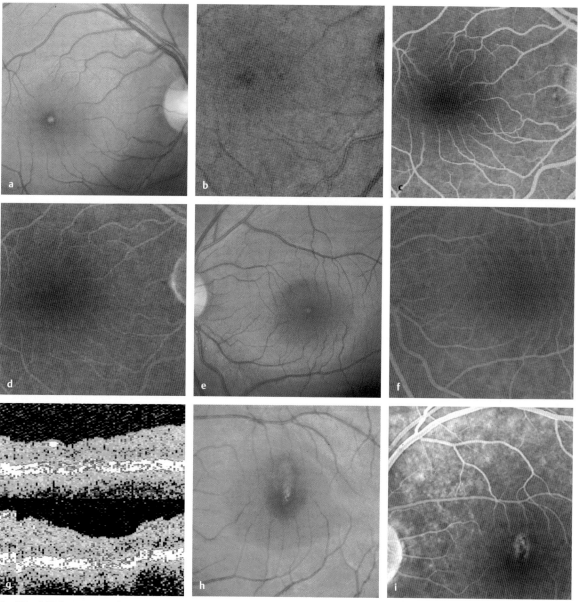

Fig. 8.7a–i Light injury to the retina

a Color photograph. Solar retinopathy, 3 days after exposure. A circular, bright lesion can still be seen in the fovea, resulting in reduced visual acuity and metamorphopsia. A completely normal fundus was seen after healing.

b Infrared image. Examination with the scanning laser ophthalmoscope indicates a clearly defined, deep lesion.

c Early arteriovenous phase. No noteworthy changes can be seen.

d Late phase. No window defects or leakages can be seen.

e Color photograph. The clinical findings in the other eye and the symptoms correspond to those in the right eye shown above.

f Late phase. No window defects or leakages are detected here either.

g Optical coherence tomography. The lower image, from the fundus shown in **a–d**, shows intraretinal edema in the acute stage, corresponding to the absence of leakage in the angiography. The upper image shows normal conditions again after healing.

h Color photograph. Solar retinopathy caused by gazing into the sun with a telescope. A scarred, clearly limited pigmentary change above the fovea can be seen after healing.

i Late arteriovenous phase. The findings are comparable to those with a laser scar. Atrophy with pigment displacement and central pigment thickening can be seen.

9.1 Toxoplasmosis Chorioretinitis   *Lothar Krause*

Epidemiology, Pathophysiology, and Clinical Presentation

- *Toxoplasma gondii* is the pathogen involved in the most common form of posterior uveitis. The infection is mainly congenitally acquired, and a scar often develops in the macular region. However, the disease can also arise in the context of postnatal toxoplasmosis infection.
- The pathogen persists in an encapsulated form in the cells. Reactivation of the pathogen can occur, and an inflammatory reaction then often appears on the edge of an old postinflammatory scar.
- On ophthalmoscopy, a yellow-white, somewhat unclear, limited retinal or chorioretinal lesion is visible, sometimes with a distinct vitreous body infiltration, which leads to a restricted view of the fundus. The acute lesions are mainly located at the posterior pole of the eye.
- An immediate juxtapapillary position (Jensen) represents a special form. A curved scotoma typically forms as a result.
- Choroidal neovascularization is a rare complication.

Fluorescein Angiography

- Fluorescein angiography is not generally necessary for diagnosis of toxoplasmosis chorioretinitis, but in certain cases it is helpful in the differential diagnosis.
- In the early phase, hypofluorescence appears in the area of the old scars, and the fresh infiltrate shows hyperfluorescence as a sign of increased leakage.
- The arteriovenous phase shows diffuse hyperfluorescence in the area of the infiltrates, and hypofluorescence appears in the region of the scars.
- In the late phase, there is an increase in the hyperfluorescence, indicating increasing leakage.

Diagnosis and Treatment

- The diagnosis is based on the ophthalmoscopic findings. Obtaining serological evidence from blood samples is often difficult. In case of uncertainty, material for a polymerase chain reaction (PCR) diagnosis can be extracted by aspirating fluid from the anterior chamber.
- The functional prognosis depends on the location of the infiltrate, with proximity to the fovea and the optic disc being the decisive aspect.
- Vasculitis, vascular occlusion, and active infiltrates can be confirmed with fluorescein angiography. Choroidal neovascularizations, as a possible complication, can also be demonstrated with this method.
- The indications for treatment vary widely. Treatment of lesions that are at a considerable distance from the optic disc and macula is not necessary, as the acute disease is self-limiting and treatment of the encapsulated form dormant in the cells is not possible.
- Treatment is required in cases in which there is an infiltration near the macular region or the optic disc. Various combinations of treatments have been described. A combination of sulfadiazine and pyrimethamine is the most common form of therapy at present (with additional systematic corticosteroid administration after an interval of 2 days).
- Clindamycin treatment is also effective, but pseudomembranous colitis can occur as a side effect in some cases.
- If choroidal neovascularization develops, treatment similar to the established regimens in age-related macular degeneration is recommended.

References

Bosch-Driessen LE, Berendschot TT, Ongkosuwito JV, Rothova A. Ocular toxoplasmosis: clinical features and prognosis of 154 patients. Ophthalmology 2002;109:869–78.

Holland GN. Ocular toxoplasmosis: new directions for clinical investigation. Ocul Immunol Inflamm 2000;8:1–7.

Holland GN, Lewis KG. An update on current practices in the management of ocular toxoplasmosis. Am J Ophthalmol 2002;134:102–14.

Mets MB, Holfels E, Boyer KM, et al. Eye manifestations of congenital toxoplasmosis. Am J Ophthalmol 1996;122:309–24.

Rothova A. Ocular manifestations of toxoplasmosis. Curr Opin Ophthalmol 2003;14:384–8.

9

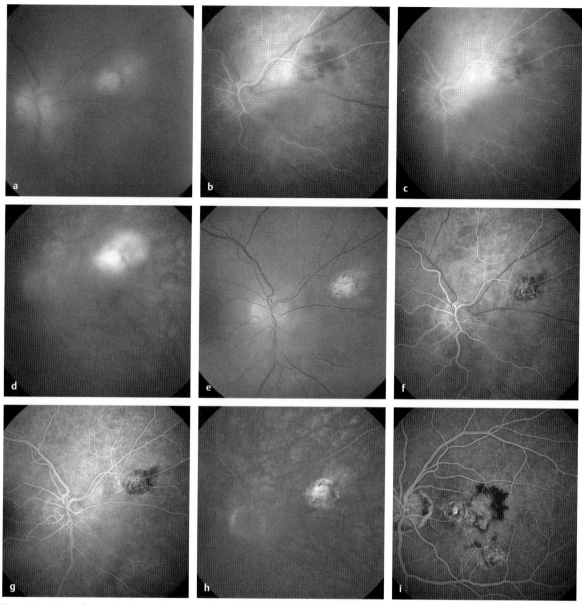

Fig. 9.1a–i Toxoplasmosis chorioretinitis

a Color photograph. At the upper temporal vessels, a whitish scar with a fleecy, inflammatory infiltrate directly adjacent to the scar is visible. The view of the fundus is restricted due to an inflammatory vitreous infiltrate.

b Early phase. Hypofluorescence in the scar area and hyperfluorescence in the acute inflamed area are visible.

c Arteriovenous phase. Incipient leakage in the border area of the scar and in the infiltrate.

d Late phase. The leakage is continuing to decrease in the scar area, as well as in the area of the fresh infiltrate.

e Color photograph. After 8 weeks of healing of the inflammatory lesion, only a scar with retinal pigment epithelial irregularities remains. There is also noticeably better visualization of the fundus.

f Early phase. Improved visibility of choroidal filling in the area of the scar.

g Arteriovenous phase. Limited hyperfluorescence in the border region of the scar.

h Late phase. The hyperfluorescence remains unchanged in the scar area.

i Arteriovenous phase (in a different patient). Choroidal neovascularization has developed at the border of a toxoplasmosis scar as a complication of the damage to the integrity of the retina, retinal pigment epithelium, and choroid.

9

9.2 Behçet Disease *Lothar Krause*

Epidemiology, Pathophysiology, and Clinical Presentation

- Behçet disease is a generalized vasculitis, with skin and mucous membrane involvement (oral and genital ulcers). The etiology is unclear, but there is probably a multifactorial pathogenesis involved a particular HLA disposition (HLA-B51) and triggering of the immune system caused by an unknown pathogen.
- Occurrences are particularly common in Asian countries.
- The retinal and choroidal vessels may be involved if there is ophthalmic involvement. Simultaneous appearance of iritis and anterior uveitis is common, but not obligatory. Hypopyon may also be present.
- Vasculitis can be found in the retina with inflammatory perivascular infiltrates and retinal hemorrhages. Vascular occlusions accompanied by ischemic areas and subsequent development of neovascularizations and secondary glaucoma can also arise.
- Acute inflammatory macular edema can progress to chronic cystoid macular edema.
- When there is optic disc involvement, swelling of the optic disc and peripapillary hemorrhage can arise, leading to optic atrophy.

Fluorescein Angiography

- Fluorescein angiography is helpful in showing the extent of the retinal ischemic areas, from mild leakages emerging from affected vessels and cystoid macular edema.
- Areas of hypofluorescence in the capillary occlusion area can be seen in the early phase, as well as ischemic areas and vessel wall irregularities.
- Areas of hyperfluorescence develop along the vessels in the arteriovenous phase due to increased permeability (involving both the arteries and the veins). Vascular occlusion and blockage of the choroidal fluorescence due to retinal and preretinal hemorrhages can be observed.
- In the late phase, hyperfluorescence intensifies due to increasing leakage, and cystoid macular edema may also become evident.

Indocyanine Green Angiography

- Indocyanine green angiography can detect additional choroidal abnormalities, particularly hypofluorescent choroidal areas after a long duration of the disease.
- The clinical relevance of these findings is questionable.

Diagnosis and Treatment

- The diagnosis is established in accordance with the criteria set out by the International Study Group for Behçet Disease: recurrent oral aphthae, plus at least two subcriteria (recurrent genital aphthae, ophthalmic involvement, skin involvement, or positive pathergy phenomenon).
- Evidence of vasculitis, vessel occlusion, ischemic areas, capillary occlusion, and cystoid macular edema can be provided by fluorescein angiography (see also Fig. 7.5 g–i).
- The treatment for ophthalmic involvement in Behçet disease includes local and/or systemic corticosteroids and immunosuppressive agents (cyclosporine, azathioprine) as basic medication to reduce the frequency of relapses.
- More recent research results have shown that the disease responds well to interferon-alpha and anti-tumor necrosis factor antibodies.

References

Atmaca LS, Batioglu F, Idil A. Retinal and disc neovascularization in Behçet's disease and efficacy of laser photocoagulation. Graefes Arch Clin Exp Ophthalmol 1996;234:94–9.

Bozzoni-Pantaleoni F, Gharbiya M, Pirraglia MP, Accorinti M, Pivetti-Pezzi P. Indocyanine green angiographic findings in Behçet disease. Retina 2001;21:230–6.

Matsuo T, Sato Y, Shiraga F, Shiragami C, Tsuchida Y. Choroidal abnormalities in Behçet disease observed by simultaneous indocyanine green and fluorescein angiography with scanning laser ophthalmoscopy. Ophthalmology 1999;106:295–300.

Stanga PE, Lim JI, Hamilton P. Indocyanine green angiography in chorioretinal diseases: indications and interpretation: an evidence-based update. Ophthalmology 2003;110:15–21.

Zouboulis CC. Epidemiology of Adamantiades–Behçet's disease. Ann Med Interne (Paris) 1999;150:488–98.

9

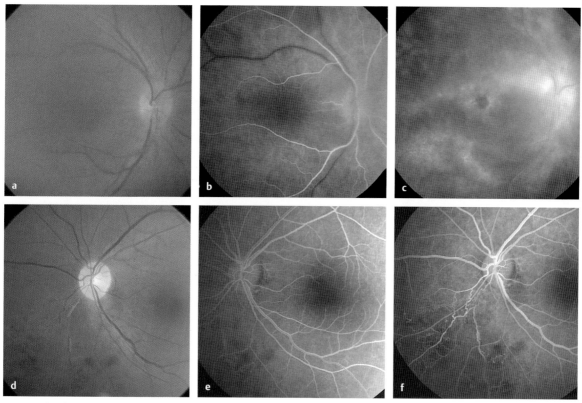

Fig. 9.2a–f Behçet disease

a Color photograph. A patient with acute inflammation in confirmed Behçet disease. The visibility of the fundus is reduced due to the inflammatory vitreous infiltrate. The macula reflex has ceased; the optic disc is lightly hyperemic.

b Early arteriovenous phase. There are discrete areas of hyperfluorescence in the paramacular area as a sign of increased permeability due to inflammation.

c Late phase. Cystoid macular edema is clearly recognizable by the parafoveal hyperfluorescence. Further areas of hyperfluorescence are visible along the temporal vessels.

d Color photograph. Dot hemorrhages, vessel occlusion, and retinal edema in the nasal lower quadrant in acute vasculitis in the context of Behçet disease.

e Arteriovenous phase. The areas of hemorrhage appear as blockage phenomena, and vascular wall irregularities are also visible. The avascular nasal lower sector appears hypofluorescent.

f Late phase. Telangiectatic vessel changes in the nasal lower quadrant. The avascular area is still hypofluorescent. Laser coagulation in the affected quadrants should be considered.

9

9.3 Cytomegalovirus and Herpes Simplex Virus Retinitis *Lothar Krause*

Cytomegalovirus Retinitis

Epidemiology, Pathophysiology, and Clinical Presentation

- Congenital cytomegalovirus transmission usually leads to a subclinical disease course. In the affected children, the illness can cause conditions ranging from hearing defects to mental retardation. The retina is involved in approximately 30% of cases.
- The acquired form of cytomegalovirus retinitis generally appears in patients receiving treatment with immunosuppressive agents and in those with acquired immune deficiency syndrome (AIDS).
- The retinitis is characterized by fluffy white retinal lesions (retinal necroses), vessel occlusions, and retinal hemorrhages.
- The retinal necroses may be extensive, and retinal detachment may occur during the course of the disease. The inflammation usually leaves behind large areas of scarring with pigment changes.

Fluorescein Angiography

- Fluorescein angiography is generally not required for diagnosis.
- Blockage phenomena develop in the early phase in the area of the hemorrhages; otherwise, proper arterial filling takes place. Vessel irregularities may occur in the affected regions.
- The arteriovenous phase shows diffuse hyperfluorescence in the area of the vessels involved and infiltrates, as well as areas of hypofluorescence due to the avascular areas.
- In the late phase, the areas of hyperfluorescence increase due to stronger and increasing leakage in the area of the inflamed vessels and possibly also in the optic disc area.

Diagnosis and Treatment

- The diagnosis is established by the ophthalmoscopic findings and the diagnostic pattern of the general findings.
- Currently, treatment consists of systematic administration of foscarnet or ganciclovir, possibly in combination with a vitreal ganciclovir implant. Therapy for possible AIDS is carried out in parallel.
- After healing of the infection, the disease course may be complicated by reactivation of the infection, or in the longer term by epiretinal gliosis, cystoid macular edema, or retinal detachment. In these cases, vitrectomy may be indicated in some circumstances.

Herpes Simplex Virus Retinitis

Epidemiology, Pathophysiology, and Clinical Presentation

- Herpes simplex virus can also be acquired either congenitally or later on. Ophthalmic involvement can lead to conjunctivitis, keratitis, or chorioretinitis. The pathogens are herpes simplex virus types I or II.
- Acute retinal necrosis in otherwise healthy individuals can occur when there is retinal involvement.
- This is characterized by extensive retinal necroses and vessel obliterations; retinal detachment may develop during the course of the disease.

Fluorescein Angiography

- Fluorescein angiography is not generally necessary for diagnosis.
- In the early phase, areas of hypofluorescence develop due to retinal and choroid vessel occlusions.
- In the arteriovenous phase, leakages develop in the area of the inflamed vessels, and hyperfluorescence in areas with edema. Hypofluorescence develops in ischemic areas and due to blockages caused by hemorrhage.
- In the late phase, increased leakage is observed.

Diagnosis and Treatment

- The diagnosis is based on the ophthalmoscopic findings.
- Treatment consists of systemic administration of acyclovir and vitreoretinal surgery if appropriate.

References

Cassoux N, Bodaghi B, Katlama C, LeHoang P. CMV retinitis in the era of HAART. Ocul Immunol Inflamm 1999;7:231–5.

Cytomegalovirus (CMV) culture results, drug resistance, and clinical outcome in patients with AIDS and CMV retinitis treated with foscarnet or ganciclovir. Studies of Ocular Complications of AIDS (SOCA) in collaboration with the AIDS Clinical Trial Group. J Infect Dis 1997;176:50–8.

Dhillon B, Ramaesh K, Leen C. Changing trends in cytomegalovirus retinitis with highly active anti-retroviral therapy (HAART). Eye 1999;13:275–6.

Goldberg DE, Wang H, Azen SP, Freeman WR. Long term visual outcome of patients with cytomegalovirus retinitis treated with highly active antiretroviral therapy. Br J Ophthalmol 2003;87:853–5.

Ritterband DC, Friedberg DN. Virus infections of the eye. Rev Med Virol 1998;8:187–201.

Tran TH, Stenescu D, Caspers-Velu L, et al. Clinical characteristics of acute HSCV-2 retinal necrosis. Am J Ophthalmol 2004;137:872–9.

9

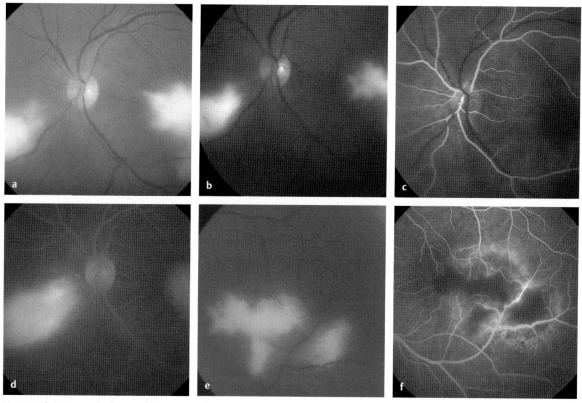

Fig. 9.3a–f Cytomegalovirus and herpes simplex virus retinitis

a Color photograph. Acute cytomegalovirus retinitis with white infiltrates located nasal and temporal to the optic disc. A vessel in the area of the nasal scars has been destroyed. The view of the fundus is reduced by cellular vitreous body infiltration.

b Black and white photograph. There are retinal infiltrates nasal and temporal to the optic disc.

c Early arteriovenous phase. There are occluded vessels in the area of the nasal infiltrates; otherwise, regular arterial filling can be seen. A filling defect is also visible in the choroid in the area of the nasal infiltrates.

d Late phase. Hyperfluorescence in the infiltrated area as an expression of increased leakage.

e Color photograph. There is a retinal infiltrate in the temporal area and vascular lesions are also present in the area of the inflamed retina.

f Arteriovenous phase. There is a filling defect (hypofluorescence) in the infiltrated area. Incipient hyperfluorescence is visible at the border of the lesion. Vascular wall irregularities and leakage from the vessels damaged by inflammation are recognizable.

9

9.4 Sarcoidosis   *Lothar Krause*

Epidemiology, Pathophysiology, and Clinical Presentation

- Sarcoidosis is a granulomatosis systemic disease, histopathologically characterized by noncaseating epithelial cellular granulomas with Langerhans giant cells. All inflammatory changes in the posterior eye should be included in the differential diagnosis of the disease.
- The etiology of sarcoidosis is not known. The disease appears most frequently in the African-American population in the USA.
- In over 90 % of cases, the disease becomes manifest in the lung (with swelling of the hilar lymph nodes), but all of the other organs can be affected in the acute or chronic forms.
- Ophthalmic involvement occurs in 25–60 % of cases. Conjunctival granuloma and chronic iridocyclitis can occur in the anterior segment. Retinal vasculitis is characterized by fluffy whitish infiltrates in the retina and perivascular infiltrations with accompanying hemorrhages. Occluded vessels may be identified. Hyperpigmentations and depigmentations develop as secondary consequences of inflammation. Retinal granulomas are rare.
- Secondary vessel proliferations are possible, due to the vessel occlusions.
- Cystoid macular edema and choroidal neovascularization may also develop.

Fluorescein Angiography

- Fluorescein angiography is useful for confirming vasculitis, vessel occlusions, active inflammatory infiltrations, cystoid macular edema, and choroidal neovascularization.
- In the early phase, areas of hyperfluorescence form along the inflamed vessels; areas of hypofluorescence arising due to capillary rarefaction and blockages arising from hyperpigmentations can also be observed.
- In the arteriovenous phase, diffuse hyperfluorescence develops in the area of the involved vessels, particularly the veins, and diffuse leakages develop in the choroid.
- The late phase shows increased hyperfluorescence due to increased leakage, and hyperfluorescence in the macular region as a possible sign of cystoid macular edema.

Indocyanine Green Angiography

- Indocyanine green angiography may show hypofluorescent lesions in the early and intermediate phases, which are irregularly distributed and not discernible on ophthalmoscopy or fluorescein angiography.
- Hyperfluorescent pinpoints may become visible in the intermediate and late phases. Fuzzy choroidal vessels with leakage in the intermediate phase and diffuse late zonal choroidal hyperfluorescence, with staining in the late phase, are also frequently observed.
- The clinical relevance of these findings is questionable.

Diagnosis and Treatment

- The diagnosis is based on the radiographic findings or computed tomography of the respiratory tract. The serum level of angiotensin-converting enzyme (ACE) is raised.
- Biopsy confirmation of the granuloma in the conjunctiva and the lung hilum is possible.
- Systemic therapy depends on the organs involved. Local administration of corticosteroids and mydriatics in the eye can be recommended. Systemic corticosteroid administration is necessary in patients with more severe ocular involvement.
- If choroidal neovascularization develops, treatment similar to the established regimens in age-related macular degeneration is recommended.

References

Dana MR, Merayo-Lloves J, Schaumberg DA, Foster CS. Prognosticators for visual outcome in sarcoid uveitis. Ophthalmology 1996; 103:1846–53.

Jabs DA, Johns CJ. Ocular involvement in chronic sarcoidosis. Am J Ophthalmol 1986;102:297–301.

Rothova A. Ocular involvement in sarcoidosis. Br J Ophthalmol 2000; 84:110–6.

Stanga PE, Lim JI, Hamilton P. Indocyanine green angiography in chorioretinal diseases: indications and interpretation: an evidence-based update. Ophthalmology 2003;110:15–21.

Stavrou P, Linton S, Young DW, Murray PI. Clinical diagnosis of ocular sarcoidosis. Eye 1997;11:365–70.

Wolfensberger TJ, Herbort CP. Indocyanine green angiographic features in ocular sarcoidosis. Ophthalmology 1999;106:285–9.

9

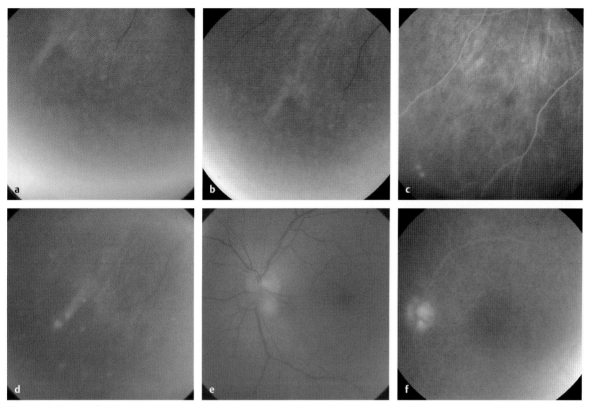

Fig. 9.**4a–f Sarcoidosis**

a Color photograph. There are whitish infiltrates located in the retinal periphery. The branched vessel clearly shows blurred edges and irregularities.

b Early phase. There is a dot-shaped hyperfluorescence on the retinal periphery. The arteries are just starting to fill.

c Arteriovenous phase. Areas of hyperfluorescence in the retinal periphery are signs of increased leakage in the areas affection by inflammation.

d Color photograph. The remaining retinal pigment epithelial defects can be identified at the site of the infiltrates after corticosteroid therapy. Fresh infiltrates are not detectable.

e Color photograph. Juxtapapillary infiltration in an acute sarcoidosis. The view of the fundus is restricted owing to vitreous opacities. The optic disc shows blurred edges, with a fluffy, whitish infiltrate at the lower edge.

f Late phase. There is mild hyperfluorescence in the optic disc as a sign of inflammatory leakage.

9.5 Posterior Scleritis   *Lothar Krause*

Epidemiology, Pathophysiology, and Clinical Presentation

- In about 40% of the cases, posterior scleritis is associated with a systemic disease (such as rheumatoid arthritis, Wegener's disease, or lupus erythematodes). The etiology often remains unknown in the remainder of the cases. Women are twice as prone to the disease as men.
- The symptoms are variable and may include pain and ocular movement disturbances. Approximately 16% of the cases are associated with a deterioration in visual acuity.
- On ophthalmoscopy, retinal changes or choroidal changes can be observed—e.g., exudative retinal detachment, choroid effusion, or choroid folds. Choroidal swelling can be so marked that it can be mistaken for choroidal melanoma.
- Optic disc swelling can be found in some cases.

Fluorescein Angiography

- The major indication for fluorescein angiography in patients with posterior scleritis is to monitor the course of the disease rather than to diagnose it, since the fluorescein-angiographic findings vary greatly.
- In the early phase, hardly any changes are visible. When there is inflammatory involvement of the choroid, finely flecked areas of hyperfluorescence may develop.
- The arteriovenous phase shows diffuse hyperfluorescence in the area of the involved choroid.
- In the late phase, an increase in the hyperfluorescence can be seen, due to continuous leakage.

Diagnosis and Treatment

- The diagnosis is based on the clinical symptoms, pain and evidence of choroidal swelling, or on ultrasound evidence of scleral changes.
- Treatment of the underlying disease is recommended. Systemic administration of nonsteroidal or corticosteroid anti-inflammatory agents is recommended in cases in which the etiology of the disease is not known.

References

Benson WE. Posterior scleritis. Surv Ophthalmol 1988;32:297–316.

Calthorpe CM, Watson PG, McCartney AC. Posterior scleritis: a clinical and histological survey. Eye 1988;2:267–77.

Demirci H, Shields CL, Honavar SG, Shields JA, Bardenstein DS. Long-term follow-up of giant nodular posterior scleritis simulating choroidal melanoma. Arch Ophthalmol 2000;118:1290–2.

McCluskey PJ, Watson PG, Lightman S, Haybittle J, Restori M, Branley M. Posterior scleritis: clinical features, systemic associations, and outcome in a large series of patients. Ophthalmology 1999;106: 2380–6.

9

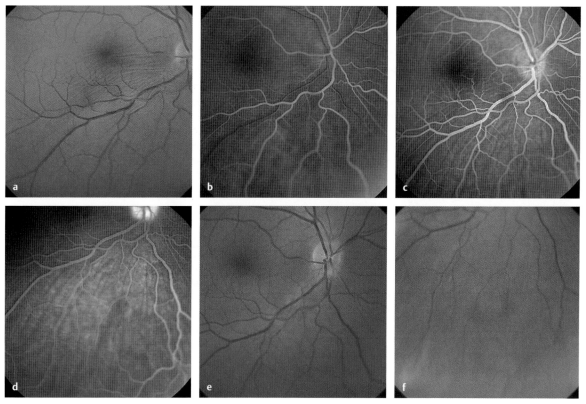

Fig. 9.**5a–f Posterior scleritis**

a Color photograph. A clear swelling of the choroid is recognizable in the temporal lower quadrant, with choroidal folds visible from the optic disc to the periphery. The optic disc and the retinal vessels appear normal.

b Early phase. Filling of the retinal arterial vessels without leakage. The retinal vessels appear blurred because of the choroidal swelling.

c Arteriovenous phase. Venous filling is normal. A streaky pattern can be seen in the choroid, without blockage to the choroidal filling.

d Late phase. The affected area has a slightly more hyperfluorescent appearance than the rest of the choroid. The streaky choroid structure is still present. In addition, fine-flecked areas of hyperfluorescence are visible in the choroid, probably representing a simultaneous inflammatory reaction.

e Color photograph. The lesions have resolved after 2 months of systemic corticosteroid therapy.

f Color photograph. No further changes are visible, even in the peripheral retina.

9.6 Vogt–Koyanagi–Harada Syndrome   *Lothar Krause*

Epidemiology, Pathophysiology, and Clinical Presentation

- Vogt–Koyanagi–Harada syndrome includes posterior uveitis in combination with inflammatory changes in the meninges, skin, or ears.
- The etiology is unknown, and the condition may be triggered by a virus. An association with the HLA-B53 antigen has been demonstrated.
- The largest number of cases occur in Asia. The age at manifestation is between 30 and 50 years. Both eyes are usually affected.
- The symptoms consist of nonspecific defects and reductions in visual acuity, headaches, meningism, fever, and dizziness.
- Hypacusis, vitiligo, and poliosis (whitening of the eyelashes) can be seen during the course of the disease.
- On biomicroscopy, anterior uveitis and chorioretinitis (which may be accompanied by exudative retinal detachment) can be seen; these can be very marked.
- The prognosis depends on the development of possible complications (cataract, glaucoma, choroidal neovascularization, and subretinal fibrotic changes). These mainly occur in patients with relapses.

Fluorescein Angiography

- Fluorescein angiography is not necessary for the diagnosis, but may be helpful in the differential diagnosis.
- In the early phase, hyperfluorescence can be identified in the inflamed choroid, with hypofluorescence flecks as a sign of circulatory dysfunction.
- In the arteriovenous phase, diffuse hyperfluorescence is present in the region of the involved retinal vessels. Later on, diffuse leakage can be found in the choroid.
- The late phase is characterized by an increase in hyperfluorescence due to increasing leakage, particularly in areas of exudative retinal detachment.

Indocyanine Green Angiography

- Indocyanine green angiography can demonstrate delayed choroidal filling, a fuzzy, indistinct appearance of the vessels in the intermediate phase, and diffuse choroidal hyperfluorescence in the late phase.
- Indocyanine green angiography may provide additional information in some cases.

Diagnosis and Treatment

- The diagnosis is based on ophthalmoscopy and the pattern of the general findings.
- Evidence of vasculitis, vascular occlusions, and active inflammatory infiltrates can be obtained with fluorescein angiography. Fluorescein angiography can also identify choroidal neovascularization as a complication.
- Therapy consists of systemic corticosteroid administration. Immunosuppressive agents may be necessary if there is no response to corticosteroid therapy.
- If choroidal neovascularization develops, treatment similar to the established regimens in age-related macular degeneration is recommended.

References

Bouchenaki N, Herbort CP: The contribution of indocyanine green angiography to the appraisal and management of Vogt–Koyanagi–Harada disease. Ophthalmology 2001;108:54–64.

Moorthy RS, Inomata H, Rao NA. Vogt–Koyanagi–Harada syndrome. Surv Ophthalmol 1995;39:265–92.

Read RW, Rao NA, Cunningham ET. Vogt–Koyanagi–Harada disease. Curr Opin Ophthalmol 2000;11:437–42.

Read RW, Rechodouni A, Butani N, et al. Complications and prognostic factors in Vogt–Koyanagi–Harada disease. Am J Ophthalmol 2001;131:599–606.

Stanga PE, Lim JI, Hamilton P. Indocyanine green angiography in chorioretinal diseases: indications and interpretation: an evidence-based update. Ophthalmology 2003;110:15–21.

9

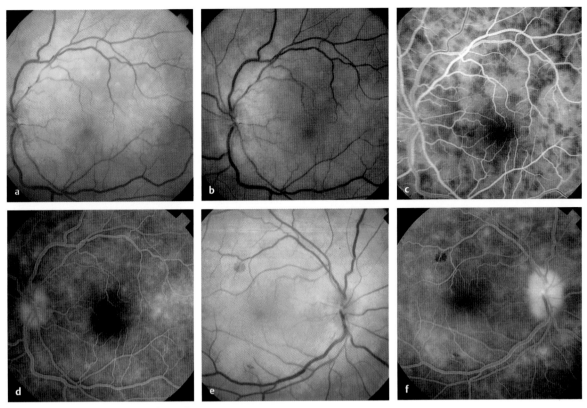

Fig. 9.6a–f Vogt–Koyanagi–Harada syndrome

a Color photograph. Serous detachment of the central retina with vessel irregularities and irregular choroidal texture.

b Early phase. There is irregular vessel filling, the vessel walls are of varying caliber, and the choroid is filling irregularly and is flecked, with clear filling defects.

c Arteriovenous phase. Fleck-shaped hypofluorescent areas in the choroid as a sign of diffuse choroiditis, with areas of filling defects and hyperfluorescence.

d Late phase. There is hyperfluorescence at the involved inflammatory optic disc, with persistence of the dot-shaped areas of choroidal hyperfluorescence.

e Color photograph. There is also a serous retinal detachment in the central area in the fellow eye, with dot-shaped hemorrhage in the temporal upper quadrant. The optic disc is swollen.

f Late phase. This eye also shows diffuse choroiditis, with fleck-shaped areas of hyperfluorescence in the choroid. The hemorrhage in the temporal upper quadrant is demarcated as a blockage. There is persistent hyperfluorescence at the optic disc.

9

9.7 Acute Posterior Multifocal Placoid Pigment Epitheliopathy   *Ulrich Kellner*

Epidemiology, Pathophysiology, and Clinical Presentation

- Acute posterior multifocal placoid pigment epitheliopathy (APMPPE) is a condition probably due to a choroidal immune vasculitis. Previous viral disease is common.
- APMPPE usually occurs in patients between 20 to 50 years of age.
- APMPPE usually affects both eyes, but the severity can differ between the eyes. The initial sign is an acute loss of visual acuity. Multiple lesions with fuzzy borders in the choroid and retinal pigment epithelium are as visible in the posterior pole as in the middle periphery of the ocular fundus. These lesions progress to more sharply delineated flecks, and later on regress to more or less marked pigmented scars.
- Spontaneous recovery usually takes place within 3–6 weeks, but relapses are possible.
- Although some of the affected eyes retain good long-term visual acuity, a persistent loss of visual acuity is possible if relapse or foveal involvement occurs.
- Choroidal neovascularization may develop as a complication.
- APMPPE has often been classified as one of the "white dot" disorders. This term refers to an ill-defined group of inflammatory disorders in which careful diagnostic work-up is needed in order to reach a specific diagnosis and decide on possible treatment.

Fluorescein Angiography

- Fluorescein angiography is useful for distinguishing between APMPPE and other choroidal diseases with fleck-like lesions.
- In the early phase, the acute APMPPE lesions are hypofluorescent due to delayed choroidal filling in the affected areas.
- Toward the late phase, distinct hyperfluorescence develops in the previously hypofluorescent lesions.
- Choroidal filling may be delayed.

Indocyanine Green Angiography

- In indocyanine green angiography, acute and older, healed lesions appear hypofluorescent during the course of the angiogram, indicating choroid hypoperfusion. This can be a helpful diagnostic sign for the differential diagnosis (see Fig. 1.**2 m–p**).

Diagnosis and Treatment

- The diagnosis is based on a combination of the ophthalmoscopic findings and fluorescein angiography.
- In optical coherence tomography, hyperreflective areas may be identified in the affected retinal pigment epithelium.
- Various inflammatory diseases of the choroid can accompany flecked lesions. Due to the frequency of the respective conditions, differential-diagnostic identification of multiple evanescent white dot syndrome (MEWDS) is important (see section 9.9). MEWDS can present with similar symptoms, and also after viral disease, but it more often occurs unilaterally and in women. Flecks also form in MEWDS, but they are generally smaller in comparison with APMPPE. The angiographic picture is also different, since in MEWDS the flecks already appear hyperfluorescent in the early stage, in contrast to the hypofluorescent flecks in APMPPE.
- There is no evidence-based treatment at present. Corticosteroid treatment has been attempted, but there is no convincing evidence that it affects the course of the disease significantly.
- If choroidal neovascularization develops, treatment similar to that in the established regimens in age-related macular degeneration is recommended.

References

Bird AC. Acute multifocal placoid pigment epitheliopathy. In: Ryan SJ, ed. Retina, 4th ed. Philadelphia, Elsevier, 2006:1803–10.

Gass JD. Acute posterior multifocal placoid pigment epitheliopathy. In: Gass JD, ed. Stereoscopic atlas of macular diseases: diagnosis and treatment, 4th ed. St. Louis: Mosby, 1997: 668–75.

Lofoco G, Giucci F, Bardocci A, et al. Optical coherence tomography findings in a case of acute multifocal posterior placoid pigment epitheliopathy (AMPPPE). Eur J Ophthalmol 2005;15:143–7.

Schneider A, Inhoffen W, Gelisken F. Indocyanine green angiography in a case of unilateral recurrent posterior acute multifocal placoid pigment epitheliopathy. Acta Ophthalmol Scand 2003;81:72–5.

Roberts TV, Mitchell P. Acute posterior multifocal placoid pigment epitheliopathy: a long-term study. Aust N Z J Ophthalmol 1997; 25:277–81.

Stanga PE, Lim JI, Hamilton P. Indocyanine green angiography in chorioretinal diseases: indications and interpretation: an evidence-based update. Ophthalmology 2003;110:15–21.

9

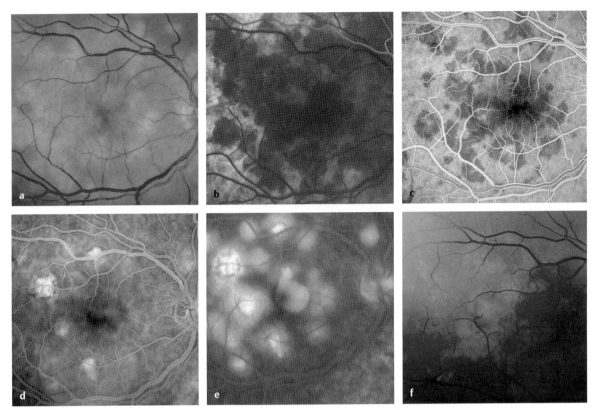

Fig. 9.**7a–f Acute posterior multifocal placoid pigment epitheliopathy**

a Color photograph. Multiple, slightly raised, partly confluent lesions can be seen at the posterior pole, extending up to the midperiphery. Fine folds are recognizable in the elevated retina around the fovea.

b Early phase. Delayed choroidal filling can be seen particularly close to the optic disc, accompanied by marked blockage in the area of the clinically visible lesions.

c Arteriovenous phase. The choroidal filling outside the acute lesions now appears to be normal; the blockage in the lesions still remains.

d Late arteriovenous phase. Incipient hyperfluorescence in the previously hypofluorescent lesions.

e Late phase. Marked hyperfluorescence in all lesions.

f Color photograph. Three months later, there is distinct, pigmented scarring of the lesions.

9.8 Birdshot Retinochoroidopathy *Ulrich Kellner*

Epidemiology, Pathophysiology, and Clinical Presentation

- Birdshot retinochoroidopathy is an autoimmune disease that is strongly associated with the antigen HLA-A29.2.
- Northern Europeans between 30 and 60 years of age are predominantly affected. The disease presents bilaterally and has a very variable course, with alternating phases of exacerbation and remission. Overall, the clinical course tends to be chronic and progressive.
- Blurred vision resulting from cystoid macular edema and floaters subsequent to vitreitis are the most common symptoms at presentation.
- Oval, whitish-yellow lesions in the outer choroid, with no initial changes in the retinal pigment epithelium, are characteristic. The lesions are often centered near the optic disc.
- Choroidal neovascularization, swelling of the optic disc, retinal vasculitis, and vitreitis can all present during the course of the disease.
- There is contradictory evidence regarding the association between birdshot retinochoroidopathy and generalized diseases. Vitiligo and vascular diseases have been reported in some studies, but not in others.
- Birdshot retinochoroidopathy has been classified as one of the "white dot" disorders. This term refers to an ill-defined group of inflammatory disorders in which careful diagnostic work-up is needed in order to reach a specific diagnosis and decide on possible treatment.

Fluorescein Angiography

- The oval lesions often present less clearly in fluorescein angiography than on ophthalmoscopy. Angiography is appropriate for diagnosing complications such as cystoid macular edema or choroidal neovascularization.
- In the early phase, the oval lesions are hypofluorescent.
- In the late phase, diffuse hyperfluorescence is often seen, due to retinal vasculitis. Cystoid macular edema may become visible.

Indocyanine Green Angiography

- Indocyanine green angiography may show dark spots between large choroidal vessels, which may be helpful in the differential diagnosis.

Diagnosis and Treatment

- The diagnosis is based on the characteristic ophthalmoscopic findings.
- Evidence of the HLA-A29.2 antigen makes the diagnosis very probable.
- Additional diagnostic tests depend on the actual symptoms. Fluorescein angiography is recommended for detection of acute vasculitis or when there is a suspicion of cystoid macular edema or choroidal neovascularization.
- Full-field electroretinography recording has been found to be helpful for monitoring the course of the disease and the success of therapeutic interventions.
- Immunosuppressive drug treatment should be administered, with or without additional corticosteroids. However, the response to the therapy is variable. Immunosuppressive drug treatment can reduce the frequency of cystoid macular edema developing.
- If choroidal neovascularization develops, treatment similar to that in the established regimens in age-related macular degeneration is recommended.
- Oral treatment with acetazolamide is useful in patients with cystoid macular edema.

References

Holder GE, Robson AG, Pavesio C, Graham EM. Electrophysiological characterization and monitoring in the management of birdshot chorioretinopathy. Br J Ophthalmol 2005;89:709–18.

Kiss S, Ahmed M, Letko E, Foster CS. Long-term follow-up of patients with birdshot retinochoroidopathy treated with corticosteroid-sparing systemic immunomodulatory therapy. Ophthalmology 2005;112:1066–71.

Levinson RD, Gonzales CR. Birdshot retinochoroidopathy: immunopathogenesis, evaluation, and treatment. Ophthalmol Clin North Am 2002;15:343–50.

Oh KT, Christmas NJ, Folk JC. Birdshot retinochoroiditis: long term follow-up of a chronically progressive disease. Am J Ophthalmol 2002;133:622–9.

Ryan SJ, Rao NA. Birdshot retinochoroidopathy. In: Ryan SJ, ed. Retina, 4th ed. Philadelphia, Elsevier, 2006:1763–70.

Stanga PE, Lim JI, Hamilton P. Indocyanine green angiography in chorioretinal diseases: indications and interpretation: an evidence-based update. Ophthalmology 2003;110:15–21.

Thorne JE, Jabs DA, Peters GB, et al. Birdshot retinochoroidopathy: ocular complications and visual impairment. Am J Ophthalmol 2005;140:45–51.

Zacks DN, Samson CM, Loewenstein J, Foster CS. Electroretinograms as an indicator of disease activity in birdshot retinochoroidopathy. Graefes Arch Clin Exp Ophthalmol 2002;240:601–7.

9

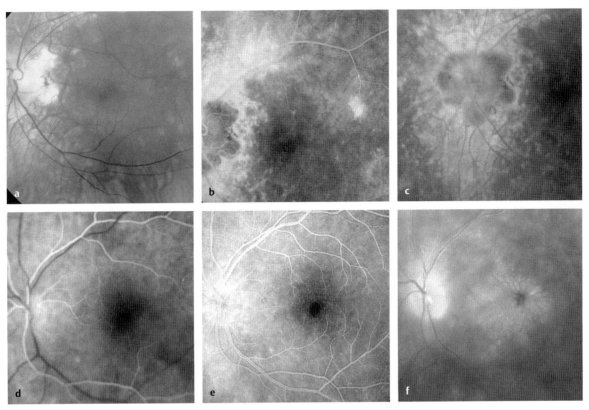

Fig. 9.8a–f Birdshot retinochoroidopathy

a Color photograph. Advanced birdshot retinochoroidopathy, with clear peripapillary atrophy.

b Arteriovenous phase. Distinct retinal pigment epithelial defects and leakage from several inflamed vessels.

c Late phase. Distinct peripapillary choriocapillaris atrophy. In this patient, progression to blindness occurred despite immunosuppressive therapy.

d Early phase (in a different patient). There is relatively normal choroidal filling, with the retinal vessels also still appearing normal.

e Arteriovenous phase. Alterations to the perifoveal capillaries have taken place, along with leakage from several of the retinal vessels.

f Late phase. Pronounced cystoid macular edema and hyperfluorescence of the inflammatory damaged vessels walls can be seen.

9.9 Multiple Evanescent White Dot Syndrome   *Ulrich Kellner*

Epidemiology, Pathophysiology, and Clinical Presentation

- Multiple evanescent white dot syndrome (MEWDS) is a rare, acute, mainly unilateral disease that is often preceded by a viral infection. An association with the HLA-B51 antigen has been suggested.
- The exact etiology is not known.
- The age of manifestation varies from 14 to 57 years of age, with women being affected more often (75% of cases).
- Patients notice an acute loss of visual acuity with photopsia; an enlarged blind spot can be detected with perimetry.
- Small, weak white flecks deep in the retina and in the retinal pigment epithelium can be seen on ophthalmoscopy, predominantly in a paramacular location at the posterior pole. The fovea also has a granular appearance.
- Vitreal cells, a blurred optic disc, and venous sheathing can also occur.
- Spontaneous recovery takes places within 3–6 weeks. Relapses are possible, but a long-term and chronic course is rare with this disease.
- Choroidal neovascularization can develop as a complication.
- MEWDS has often been classified as one of the "white dot" disorders. This term refers to an ill-defined group of inflammatory disorders in which careful diagnostic work-up is needed in order to reach a specific diagnosis and decide on possible treatment.
- In addition, on the basis of the overlapping of clinical signs in several rare (and acronym-prone) retinochoroidal inflammatory disorders, there is ongoing discussion on whether MEWDS, acute idiopathic blind spot enlargement syndrome (AIBSE), punctate inner choroidopathy (PIC), multifocal inner choroiditis (MIC or MFIC), acute macular neuroretinitis (AMN), and acute zonal occult outer retinopathy (AZOOR) are different conditions with a similar pathogenesis or whether they constitute separate entities. It will only be possible to decide the issue when the etiology of each of these disorders is better defined.

Fluorescein Angiography

- Fluorescein angiography is useful for distinguishing MEWDS from other choroidal diseases with fleck-like lesions.
- In the early phase, the clinically visible lesions present as dot-like areas of hyperfluorescence.
- Hyperfluorescence of the lesions persists in the late phase. In addition, diffuse fleck-shaped leakage can emerge in the retinal pigment epithelium, from the retinal vessels, or from the capillaries of the optic disc.
- Following regression of the acute lesions, window defects in the retinal pigment epithelium may persist.

Indocyanine Green Angiography

- Hypofluorescent lesions are present up to the late stages of indocyanine green angiography (ICG), indicating choroidal vascular abnormalities.
- Hypofluorescent areas on ICG angiography correspond to visual field defects. During regression, hypofluorescent areas persist, indicating persistent choroidal vascular damage, although the visual fields in these areas improve.

Diagnosis and Treatment

- The diagnosis of multiple evanescent white dot syndrome is established on the basis of the clinical findings and angiography. Differentiation between acute posterior multifocal placoid pigment epitheliopathy (APMPPE; see section 9.7) is based on the size of the lesions and the different appearance of the lesions in the early stage of angiography. They are hypofluorescent in APMPPE and hyperfluorescent in MEWDS.
- An enlarged blind spot and also small scotomas are often found in perimetry.
- Functional analyses and specific electrophysiological tests (early receptor potential) can suggest a dysfunction in the cone–pigment epithelium complex. However, these tests are generally not necessary for clinical diagnosis.
- There is at present no available treatment.
- If choroidal neovascularization develops, treatment similar to the established regimens in age-related macular degeneration is recommended.

References

Francis PJ, Marinescu A, Fitzke FW, Bird AC, Holder GE. Acute zonal occult outer retinopathy: towards a set of diagnostic criteria. Br J Ophthalmol 2005;89:70–3.

Gass JD. Multiple evanescent white dot syndrome. In: Gass JD, ed. Stereoscopic atlas of macular diseases: diagnosis and treatment, 4th ed. St. Louis: Mosby, 1997: 678–81.

Ikeda N, Ikeda T, Nagata M, et al. Location of lesions in multiple evanescent white dot syndrome and the cause of hypofluorescent spots observed by indocyanine green angiography. Graefes Arch Clin Exp Ophthalmol 2001;239:242–7.

Stanga PE, Lim JI, Hamilton P. Indocyanine green angiography in chorioretinal diseases: indications and interpretation: an evidence-based update. Ophthalmology 2003;110:15–21.

Tsai L, Jampol LM. Multiple evanescent white-dot syndrome. In: Ryan SJ, ed. Retina, 4th ed. Philadelphia, Elsevier, 2006:1785–92.

Yen MT, Rosenfeld PJ. Persistent indocyanine green angiographic findings in multiple evanescent white dot syndrome. Ophthalmic Surg Lasers 2001;32:156–8.

9

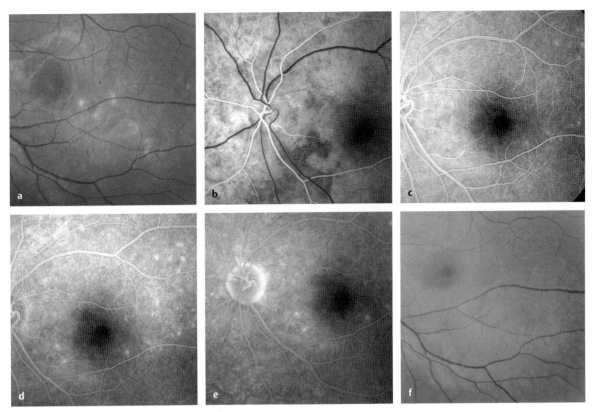

Fig. 9.9a–f Multiple evanescent white dot syndrome

a Color photograph. Multiple small fleck-like lesions are visible, particularly temporal to the fovea.

b Early phase. There is irregular choroidal filling, and the flecks are not yet visible.

c Arteriovenous phase. The lesions show various degrees of hyperfluorescence.

d Late arteriovenous phase. Persistent hyperfluorescence, with no increase.

e Late phase. Persistent hyperfluorescence, with no increase.

f Color photograph. After 5 months, the lesions have completely disappeared.

9

9.10 Serpiginous Choroiditis   *Ulrich Kellner*

Epidemiology, Pathophysiology, and Clinical Presentation

- Serpiginous choroiditis (also known as geographic choroiditis and helicoid peripapillary choroidopathy) is a bilateral, chronic, and recurrent choroidal disease with an unclear pathogenesis.
- The symptoms usually become manifest between 40 and 60 years of age.
- Relatively clearly defined, gray-white acute lesions develop in the choroid and in the retinal pigment epithelium, starting near the optic disc. The initial stages are generally asymptomatic, so that when subjective symptoms develop, new lesions can usually be seen bordering or adjacent to older scars.
- Regression of an acute lesion leads to a chorioatrophic scar. Choroidal neovascularization occurs with a frequency of up to 25%.
- The individual symptoms at presentation mainly depend on the degree of parafoveal and foveal involvement either by inflammatory lesions or choroidal neovascularization.
- Helicoid peripapillary chorioretinal dystrophy, a very rare condition with autosomal-dominant inheritance, is a differential diagnosis in patients who do not have acute inflammation.
- Serpiginous choroiditis has often been classified as one of the "white dot" disorders. This term refers to an ill-defined group of inflammatory disorders in which careful diagnostic work-up is needed in order to reach a specific diagnosis and decide on possible treatment.

Fluorescein Angiography

- Angiography is of limited value in the diagnostic work-up, as both the atrophic scars and the acute lesions are generally recognizable clinically. A partly regressed lesion may be more easy to detect on fluorescein angiography.
- Hypofluorescent lesions and blockages can be found in the early phase.
- During the course of the angiogram, increasing hyperfluorescence is observed in the acute lesions.
- Distinct choriocapillaris defects are present during the scar stage. Hypofluorescence is visible in the scars themselves, and staining can be found on the edge of the scars in the late phase.

Indocyanine Green Angiography

- Indocyanine green angiography shows well-defined hypofluorescent lesions up to the late phase.

Diagnosis and Treatment

- The ophthalmoscopic findings are usually characteristic, so that no further diagnostic measures are necessary apart from taking a family history to exclude the possibility of dominant helicoid peripapillary chorioretinal dystrophy.
- Angiography may be helpful for identifying acute lesions and differentiating inflammatory lesions from choroidal neovascularization.
- There is limited experience with the few treatment options available. Immunosuppressive drugs and alkylating agents have shown potential benefits in small series. Intravitreal administration of corticosteroids and interferon alpha have been beneficial in individual cases. Due to the rareness of the disease, it is difficult to carry out large-scale studies on the efficacy of treatment. Due to the poor prognosis with the natural course of the disease, an attempt at treatment would appear to be justified for these patients.
- If choroidal neovascularization develops, treatment similar to the established regimens in age-related macular degeneration is recommended. This treatment has no effect on the course of the choroidopathy.

References

Christmas NJ, Oh KT, Oh DM, Folk JC. Long-term follow-up of patients with serpiginous choroiditis. Retina 2002;22:550–6.

Gass JD. Serpiginous choroiditis (geographic choroiditis, helicoid peripapillary choroidopathy). In: Gass JD, ed. Stereoscopic atlas of macular diseases: diagnosis and treatment, 4th ed. St. Louis: Mosby, 1997: 158–65.

Jumper MJ, McDonald HR, Johnson RN, Ai E, Fu AD. Serpiginous Choroiditis. In: Ryan SJ, ed. Retina, 4th ed. Philadelphia, Elsevier, 2006:1811–20.

Lim WK, Buggage RR, Nussenblatt RB: Serpiginous choroiditis. Surv Ophthalmol 2005;50:231–44.

Stanga PE, Lim JI, Hamilton P. Indocyanine green angiography in chorioretinal diseases: indications and interpretation: an evidence-based update. Ophthalmology 2003;110:15–21.

9

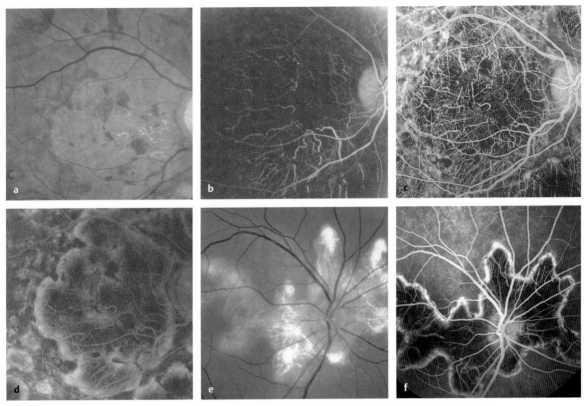

Fig. 9.**10a–f Serpiginous choroiditis**

a Color photograph. There are distinct, sometimes circumscribed but mainly confluent areas of chorioatrophic scarring at the posterior pole.

b Early phase. Clear filling of the large choroidal vessel in the absence of choriocapillaris and retinal pigment epithelium.

c Middle phase. The large choroidal vessels are visible.

d Late phase. Scar staining at the edge of the lesions.

e Color photograph. There are finger-shaped chorioatrophic scars fanning out form the optic disc.

f Late phase. Clear staining on the edge of the scars.

9

10.1 Differential Diagnosis in Optic Disc Swelling and Anterior Ischemic Optic Neuropathy *Claudia Jandeck*

Optic Disc Swelling

- The causes of optic disc swelling can rarely be clearly diagnosed by ophthalmoscopy alone. Usually, the etiology has to be deduced from the case history, accompanying symptoms, and additional diagnostic methods.
- Optic disc swelling can be caused by any of the following disorders, for example:
  - Anterior ischemic optic neuropathy (AION), arteritic or nonarteritic
  - Inflammation due to autoimmune reactions (e.g., optic neuritis, sarcoidosis, or uveitis) or due to infection (e.g., toxoplasmosis, borreliosis, and syphilis)
  - Intracranial hypertension (papilledema)
  - Tumors (glioma, meningioma, orbital tumors)
  - Anomalies (optic disc drusen, hyperopia)
  - Rare: Leber's congenital amaurosis, radiation optic neuropathy, ocular hypotony, side effects of drugs
- Fluorescein angiography is helpful in the diagnostic work-up only when the findings are clear. Examples with classic findings are presented in this chapter.

Anterior Ischemic Optic Neuropathy

Epidemiology, Pathophysiology, and Clinical Presentation

- Anterior ischemic optic neuropathy (AION) is the most common form of optic disc swelling.
- Reduced circulation in the shorter ciliary arteries is caused in two-thirds of cases by arteriosclerotic changes, and in one-third by inflammation. Circulatory dysfunction can develop anterior to, inside, or just behind the lamina cribrosa.
- Reduced perfusion pressure and an acute lack of oxygen then lead to anterior ischemic optic neuropathy, with optic disc swelling caused by blockage of the fast axoplasmic flow.

Nonarteritic Form

- The incidence is one in 10 000 in the general population and 2–10 per 100 000 per year in those over the age of 50. The fellow eye is affected in approximately 19% of cases within 5 years. Men and women are equally at risk.
- Risk factors are arterial hypertension in 49% of cases and diabetes mellitus in 26%. Other risk factors include sleep apnea syndrome, cardiovascular or cerebrovascular diseases, carotid changes, coagulation dysfunction, and optic disc hypoplasia.
- A sudden unilateral decrease in visual acuity is often experienced (42%) within the first 2 hours after waking. Patients present with visual acuity loss, abnormal color vision, visual field defects (the inferior visual field is affected in 47% of cases), and optic disc swelling.

Arteritic Form (Caused by Arteritis Temporalis, Giant-Cell Arteritis, Horton Disease)

- The incidence is 15–30 per 100 000 per year in those over the age of 50. Without treatment, the fellow eye is affected within a few days in 95% of cases. Women are more often affected than men (3 : 1).
- The typical case history consists of temporal headache and jaw claudication. Double vision, abnormal fatigue, subfebrile temperatures and polymyalgia rheumatica are less frequent.
- Clinically, optic disc swelling, a distinct reduction in visual acuity, tenderness and absent pulsation in the temporal artery, and an increase in the erythrocyte sedimentation rate (ESR) and C-reactive protein (CRP) level are observed. However, the ESR may be normal in up to 20% of the patients.

10

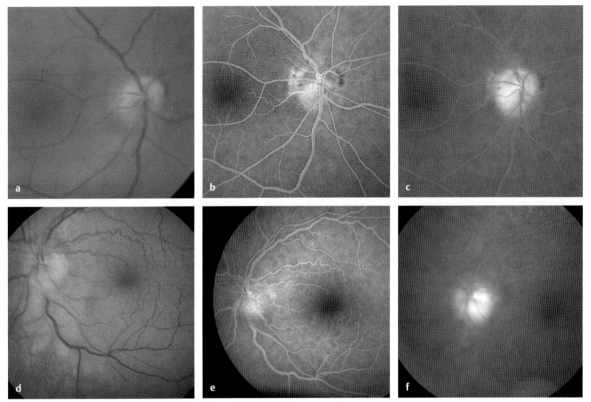

Fig. 10.1a–f   Differential diagnosis in optic disc swelling and anterior ischemic optic neuropathy

a Color photograph. Anterior ischemic optic neuropathy, with mild optic disc swelling. The optic disc swelling is more noticeable below than above (segmental). Individual areas of hemorrhage are visible in the temporal area on the edge of the optic disc.

b Arteriovenous phase. There is a filling delay in the optic disc, with a minimal delay in peripapillary choroidal filling.

c Late phase. The leakage remains limited to the optic disc.

d Color photograph. Anterior ischemic optic neuropathy: the optic disc is prominent, with indistinct borders.

e Arteriovenous phase. There is a filling delay at the top in the optic disc and incipient leakage.

f Late phase. The leakage remains limited to the optic disc.

10

Inflammatory Anterior Ischemic Optic Neuropathy

- Anterior ischemic optic neuropathy can develop due to infection or as a parainfectious finding in association with borreliosis, chlamydiosis, *Mycoplasma* infection, neurotropic viruses, and paraneoplastic inflammation.

Clinical Findings for All Forms

- The optic disc often shows focal nerve fiber hemorrhages, diffuse or focal telangiectasis, and sectorial or diffuse swelling. Narrowing of the arteries on the optic disc may also be seen.
- Hard exudates are occasionally present in peripapillary area or in the macula.
- Resorption of optic disc swelling takes place within 4–8 weeks. Segmental or diffuse paleness appears after resorption.

Fluorescein Angiography

- A delay in filling of the optic disc area and possibly a nominal delay in peripapillary choroidal filling occur in the early phase.
- In the later phases, leakage takes place at the optic disc and is limited to that area.

Diagnosis and Treatment

- The diagnostic work-up includes visual acuity, visual field examination, monitoring of eye mobility (for findings such as double vision or movement pain), and ESR and CRP assessment.
- For differential diagnosis, temporal artery biopsy, Doppler sonography, computed tomography or magnetic resonance imaging (if there is no regression of optic disc swelling), and a check for inflammatory or neoplastic systemic diseases can be carried out.
- It is important to exclude possible cardiovascular risk factors (long-term electrocardiography, transesophageal echocardiography). It is also important to exclude autoimmune diseases, particularly in younger patients.

Nonarteritic Anterior Ischemic Optic Neuropathy

- It is important to treat the underlying disease and risk factors (diabetes mellitus, hypertension).
- Acetylsalicylic acid (ASA) 100 mg/d can be administered for prophylactic treatment (preferably short-term rather than long-term).
- It is not yet clear whether treatments with isovolemic hemodilution in the acute phase, early administration of anticoagulants, or the administration of levodopa are effective.
- Vasoconstrictive agents (e. g., ergotamine for migraine or nasal sprays) should be avoided.
- Visual acuity improves in 10–35 % of cases, and relapses are rare.

Arteritic Anterior Ischemic Optic Neuropathy

- Immediate hospital admission for high-dose treatment with corticosteroids (500–1000 mg prednisone equivalent i. v.; two to four single doses per day) is necessary.
- Corticosteroid administration is reduced with repeated ESR testing. Long-term administration of low-dose corticosteroids is necessary.
- Improvement in visual acuity is rare.

References

Buono LM, Foroozan R, Sergott RC, Savino PJ. Nonarteritic anterior ischemic optic neuropathy. Curr Opin Ophthalmol 2002;13:357–61.

Ghanchi FD, Dutton GN. Current concepts in giant cell (temporal) arteritis. Surv Ophthalmol 1997;42:99–123.

Hattenauer MG, Leavitt JA, Hotge DO, Grill R, Gray DT. Incidence of nonarteritic anterior ischemic optic neuropathy. Am J Ophthalmol 1997;123:103–7.

Ischemic Optic Neuropathy Decompression Trial Research Group. Optic nerve decompression surgery for nonarteritic ischemic optic neuropathy (NAION) is not effective and may be harmful. JAMA 1995;273:625–32.

10

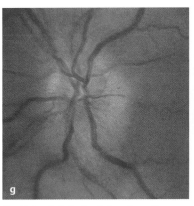
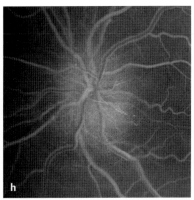
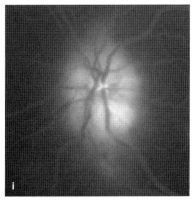

Fig. 10.**1g–i Anterior ischemic optic neuropathy**

g Color photograph. Anterior ischemic optic neuropathy. The swollen optic disc has indistinct borders.

h Early phase. There is mild leakage in the area of the optic disc, with minimal filling delay in the upper temporal area. Dilated capillaries are recognizable on the optic disc.

i Late phase. The leakage remains limited to the optic disc.

10.2 Optic Neuritis *Claudia Jandeck*

Epidemiology, Pathophysiology, and Clinical Presentation

- Various diseases have to be distinguished from optic neuritis in the differential diagnosis.
- The most common is optic neuritis caused by autoimmune conditions (with an incidence of five per 100 000 per year). There is a 22% likelihood of multiple sclerosis developing within 10 years if no white-matter lesions are evident on magnetic resonance imaging (MRI). The risk increases to 56% if at least one white-matter lesion is present.
- Other autoimmune processes causing optic neuritis include vasculitis, sarcoidosis, lupus erythematosus, panarteritis nodosa, and Crohn disease.
- Inflammatory causes include toxoplasmosis, borreliosis, syphilis, herpes zoster, and parainfectious processes.
- Toxic causes include side effects of drugs and radiation optic neuropathy.
- Generally, a slow (within days) unilateral decrease in visual acuity develops, and eye movement is painful in 92% of cases.
- Visual impairment increases as the body temperature rises.
- A central scotoma develops in the visual field. There is a latency delay in the pattern visual evoked potential (VEP).
- Ophthalmoscopically, a swollen and prominent optic disc can be seen. Hemorrhages at the optic disc are rare.
- Swelling of the retrobulbar optic nerve can be demonstrated with ultrasonography.

Fluorescein Angiography

- Fluorescein angiography is not necessary for diagnostic purposes. As optic neuritis can be associated with various diseases, familiarity with the findings is important when assessing the angiographic images.
- Early leakage of dye from the dilated capillaries takes place in the early phase.
- Accentuated hyperfluorescence appears in the prominent optic disc areas in the arteriovenous phase.
- The leakage remains restricted to the optic disc in the late phase.

Diagnosis and Treatment

- The diagnosis is based on the typical case history and ophthalmoscopic findings.
- Pattern VEP is important for follow-up and for examination of the fellow eye.
- MRI of the brain and a neurological examination should be carried out for further clarification.
- A serological analysis can be undertaken to clarify the differential diagnosis.
- The prognosis and treatment depend on the cause of the optic neuritis.
- Treatment of optic neuritis is advisable if demyelinating lesions are evident on MRI or the patient is severely affected by reduced visual acuity:
  - Days 1–3: 4 × 250 g methylprednisolone as a short infusion
  - Days 4–14: 1 mg/kg body weight prednisone orally
  - Day 15: 20 mg prednisone orally
  - Days 16–18: 10 mg prednisone orally
- Combination treatment with immunomodulating agents may be even more promising in order to reduce the risk of multiple sclerosis developing later.
- The prognosis for the recovery of visual acuity is relatively good. After 1 month, visual acuity is 1.0 in 65% of the patients and at least 0.5 in 95% of the patients.
- Irreversible damage generally develops with other autoimmune processes. Early steroid therapy and, depending on the diagnosis, additional specific general therapy is recommended.

References

Arnold AC. Evolving management of optic neuritis and multiple sclerosis. Am J Ophthalmol 2005;139:1101–8.

Beck RW. Clinically definite multiple sclerosis following optic neuritis. Ann Neurol 1997;42:815–6.

Beck RW, Trobe JD. The Optic Neuritis Treatment Trial. Putting the results in perspective. The Optic Neuritis Study Group. J Neuroophthalmol 1995;15:131–5.

Beck RW, Trobe JD, Moke PS, et al. High- and low-risk profiles for the development of multiple sclerosis within 10 years after optic neuritis: experience of the Optic Neuritis Treatment Trial. Arch Ophthalmol 2003;121:944–9.

10

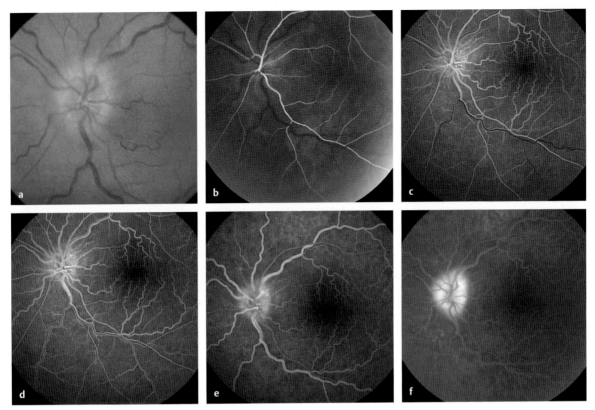

Fig. 10.2a–f   Optic neuritis

a   Color photograph. Swelling of the optic disc in optic neuritis.

b   Early phase. There is early leakage of dye from the dilated capillaries.

c   Early arteriovenous phase. Hyperfluorescence is visible in the prominent disc areas.

d   Arteriovenous phase. The hyperfluorescence is increasing.

e   Late phase. There is clear leakage in the area of the optic disc.

f   Late phase. The leakage remains limited to the optic disc.

10.3 Optic Nerve Head Anomalies   *Claudia Jandeck*

Myelinated Retinal Nerve Fibers (Fibrae Medullares)

Epidemiology, Pathophysiology, and Clinical Presentation

- This developmental anomaly is found in < 1% of ophthalmology patients. It is bilateral in 20% of cases, and men are more often affected than women.
- The condition is caused by myelinated axons of the retinal ganglion cells in the optic nerve and retina areas. Myelination occasionally extends past the lamina cribrosa along the nerve fibers of the optic nerve head and the sensory retina.
- There is an association with the triad of amblyopia, strabismus, and myopia.
- Sector-shaped or flame-shaped whitish or gray-white areas can usually be seen originating from the optic disc and accompanying the nerve fibers. Because of the uneven length of the myelin sheaths, there is a characteristic feathered appearance on the edge. Small areas of myelinated nerve fibers remote from the optic disc are a less frequent finding.
- The retinal vessels may be completely or partially obscured as a result of the myelinated retinal nerve fibers.
- Ophthalmoscopically, the myelin sheaths surrounding the nerve fibers of the optic disc and retina have an opaque white appearance.

Fluorescein Angiography

- The myelinated nerve fibers show discrete hypofluorescence due to blockage of choroidal fluorescence in all phases of the angiography. Hyperfluorescence is not observed.

Diagnosis and Treatment

- The typical clinical findings require the exclusion or treatment of possible amblyopia, strabismus, and myopia. Fluorescein angiography is only needed to establish the diagnosis in exceptional cases.
- The area of myelinated nerve fibers remains unchanged throughout the patient's life and does not require any specific treatment.
- Rarely, changes in the myelination have been observed after radiation therapy and in other retinal disorders.

References

Gicquel JJ, Salama B, Mercie M, et al. Myelinated retinal nerve fibres loss in Leber's hereditary optic neuropathy. Acta Ophthalmol Scand 2005;83:517–8.

Lee MS, Gonzalez C. Unilateral peripapillary myelinated retinal nerve fibers associated with strabismus, amblyopia, and myopia. Am J Ophthalmol 1998;125:554–6.

Mashayekhi A, Shields CL, Shields JA. Disappearance of retinal myelinated nerve fibers after plaque radiotherapy for choroidal melanoma. Retina 2003;23:572–3.

Straatsma BR, Foos RY, Heckenlively JR, Taylor GN. Myelinated retinal nerve fibers. Am J Ophthalmol 1981;91:25–38.

Optic Nerve Pits

Epidemiology, Pathophysiology, and Clinical Presentation

- The incidence is congenital and sporadic (one in 11 000) and is bilateral in 15% of cases. In 95% of cases, only one pit is present in the temporal area.
- The condition is caused by an occlusion defect in the embryonic ventral fissure of the optic nerve.
- There are associations with other malformations such as Aicardi syndrome, CHARGE syndrome (coloboma of the eye, heart anomaly, choanal atresia, retardation, and genital and ear anomalies), orbital cysts, congenital forebrain malformations, basal encephalocele, and absent corpus callosum.
- Morning glory syndrome is an extremely large optic disc with a tunnel-shaped excavation and distinct peripapillary pigmentation.
- The pit size ranges from 0.1 to 0.7 optic disc diameters and has a depth ranging from 0.5–2.5 D. In color, the pits may be gray (60%), yellow (30%), or black (10%). The border may be raised as a result of pigment changes (95%).
- Visual field defects are observed in 60% of cases and reduced visual acuity in 7%, mainly due to exudative macular detachment.

Fluorescein Angiography

- Fluorescein angiography does not have any diagnostic relevance, but can be used to assess the extent of the exudative retinal detachment.

Diagnosis and Treatment

- The diagnosis is based on the clear clinical findings. Optical coherence tomography can also be helpful.
- Magnetic resonance imaging is also recommended in order to eliminate cerebral changes, and internal-medicine and neurological examinations are recommended in order to exclude associated syndromes.
- Temporal pits can lead to exudative retinal detachment in 50% of cases in young patients. Surgical treatments for persistent macular detachment include photocoagulation and vitrectomy using gas tamponade and/or autologous platelet concentrate.

References

Bartz-Schmidt KU, Heimann K, Esser P. Vitrectomy for macular detachment associated with optic nerve pits. Int Ophthalmol 1995;19:323–9.

Hornby SJ, Adolph S, Gilbert CE, Dandona CE, Foster A. Visual acuity in children with coloboma: clinical features and a new phenotype classification system. Ophthalmology 2000;107:511–20.

Johnson TM, Johnson MW. Pathogenic implications of subretinal gas migration through pits and atypical colobomas of the optic nerve. Arch Ophthalmol 2004;122:1793–800.

Poulson AV, Snead DR, Jacobs PM, Ahmad N, Snead MP. Intraocular surgery for optic nerve disorders. Eye 2004;18:1056–65.

Ruthlege BK, Puliafito CA, Duker JS, Hee MR, Cox MS. Optical coherence tomography of macular lesions associated with optic nerve head pits. Ophthalmology 1996;103:1047–53.

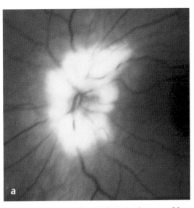
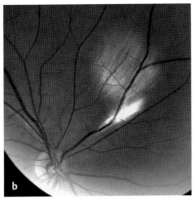
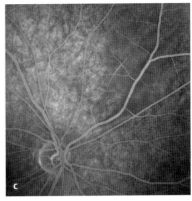

Fig. 10.**3a–c Myelinated retinal nerve fibers (fibrae medullares)**

a Color photograph in myelinated nerve fibers. There are whitish myelinated nerve fibers with irregular borders.

b Red-free image. Myelinated nerve fibers are visible remote from the optic disc.

c Late phase. There is discrete hypofluorescence in the myelinated nerve fibers area, with no leakage or accumulation of dye throughout the whole angiography.

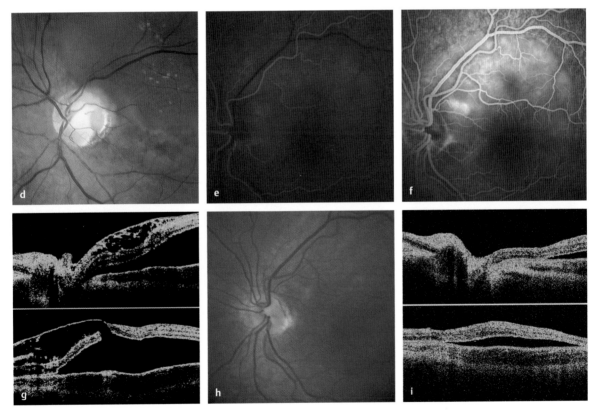

Fig. 10.**3d–i Optic nerve pits**

d Color photograph. There is an optic nerve pit in the temporal disc area, with adjacent exudative retinal detachment.

e Early stage (different patient). Mild hyperfluorescence indicating leakage in the area of serous retinal detachment associated with a temporal optic nerve pit. The patient had noted visual loss for about 8 months (visual acuity 0.2).

f Arteriovenous stage. Increased leakage in the area of serous retinal detachment.

g Optical coherence tomography (OCT) of the optic disc (upper image) and macula (lower image). A subretinal space reaches from the optic disc to the macula under the detached retina. In addition, inner retinal edematous alterations are seen between optic disc and fovea. These images were taken prior to vitreoretinal surgery with gas tamponade.

h Color photography (same patient as **e–g**). Seven months after vitreoretinal surgery ophthalmoscopically the retina appears to be attached, visual acuity has improved to 0.4.

i OCT of the optic disc (upper image) and macula (lower image). The area of retinal detachment has considerably decreased in size. No connection between macular detachment and optic disc persists. The inner retinal edematous lesions have disappeared as well.

Optic Disc Drusen _____

Epidemiology, Pathophysiology, and Clinical Presentation

- The incidence is 10–20 per 1000 in histological studies and three per 1000 in clinical studies.
- Drusen are bilateral in 69–73% of cases. They are probably already present at birth and are first clinically observed at the age of six.
- They are more common in patients with retinitis pigmentosa and angioid streaks.
- Drusen of the optic disc consist of hyaline bodies, are often partly calcified, and are located anterior to the lamina cribrosa. They develop due to an abnormal intracellular metabolism with calcification of the mitochondria.
- Four different types can be distinguished:
  - Associated with acquired diseases (hypertension, vessel occlusion, chorioretinitis)
  - Associated with hereditary degenerative diseases (phacomatoses)
  - Idiopathic (usually with autosomal-dominant inheritance)
  - Simple giant drusen
- Visual field defects are nonspecific. Reduced visual acuity is possible as a result of the growth of the drusen, with pressure on the axons and subsequent partial optic atrophy.
- Transient amaurosis (ranging from seconds to hours) may occur.
- A narrow scleral canal, a prominent optic disc, and possibly dilated capillaries are clinically visible. Hemorrhage on the edge of the optic disc occurs in 14% of cases and shunt vessels in 7% of cases. Rarely, juxtapapillary subretinal hemorrhage occurs.

Fluorescein Angiography

- Fluorescein angiography is only beneficial for identifying additional vascular changes and choroidal neovascularization.

Diagnosis and Treatment

- In ophthalmoscopy, the diagnosis is based on illumination of the drusen.
- The drusen can generally only be observed with autofluorescence if they are also visible ophthalmoscopically.
- Ultrasonography (B-imaging) also makes it possible to identify deep-lying drusen. A negative finding does not exclude the diagnosis in children or young adults.
- It is helpful to examine other family members as well.
- Computed tomography is recommended if the differential diagnosis is unclear.
- Risk factors or accompanying diseases should be clarified before the final diagnosis.
- There is no treatment for optic disc drusen. Treatment may be necessary for secondary changes such as choroidal neovascularization.
- The long-term prognosis is relatively good in the majority of patients.

References

Auw-Haedrich C, Staubach F, Witschel H. Optic disc drusen. Surv Ophthalmol 2002;47:515–32.

Friedman AH, Beckermann B, Gold DH, et al. Drusen of the optic disc. Surv Ophthalmol 1977;21:375–90.

Glaser JS. Topical diagnosis: prechiasmal pathways. Part II: the optic nerve. In: Tasman W, Jaeger EA, eds. Duane's clinical ophthalmology, vol. 2. Philadelphia: Lippincott Williams and Wilkins, 1999: 35–7.

Lorentzen SE. Drusen of the optic disc: a clinical and genetic study. Acta Ophthalmol Suppl 1966;90:1–181.

Tso MO. Pathology and pathogenesis of drusen of the optic nerve head. Ophthalmology 1981;88:1066–80.

10

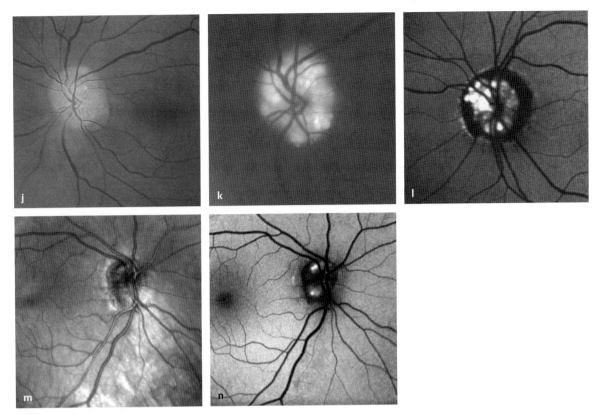

Fig. 10.**3j–n Optic disc drusen**

j Color photograph. Multiple prominent drusen are visible in the optic disc.

k Late phase. There is hyperfluorescence without leakage.

l Fundus autofluorescence (in a different patient). Autofluorescence is visible in several drusen.

m Infrared imaging (in a different patient). Prominence of the optic disc is visible.

n Fundus autofluorescence: Autofluorescence of several drusen are present in the optic disc.

10.4 Papilledema   *Claudia Jandeck*

Epidemiology, Pathophysiology, and Clinical Presentation

- Papilledema occurs if the intracranial pressure (normally 3–15 mmHg) is higher than the intraocular pressure.
- Papilledema is generally bilateral.
- Unilateral papilledema may be observed in patients with tumors of the optic nerve—e. g., meningioma or glioma; or in those with external compression of the optic nerve—e. g., endocrine orbitopathy (muscle swelling), ethmoidal cysts, and retrobulbar tumors.
- Slow axoplasmic flow is blocked at the level of the lamina cribrosa and accumulates in front of it. Swelling of the axons takes place, with edema developing and consequently leading to peripheral dislocation of the retinal cells. This causes enlargement of the blind spot.
- The symptoms can include foggy vision, cloudy vision, reduced visual acuity, and sixth nerve palsy. Amaurosis fugax (caused by standing up) is observed is some cases. Exophthalmos (due to retrobulbar expansion) may also be present.
- Headaches, vomiting, cramp, respiratory disturbances, and psychological changes occur with intracranial pressure.
- Papilledema is classified into five stages in accordance with the Frisen scheme.
- In the early stage, the optic disc changes include: minimal hyperemia, discrete swelling of the nerve fibers, and an absent spontaneous vein pulse. Additional clinical findings in the more advanced stages are: marked optic disc prominence, enlarged diameter, circumferential halo, vessel tortuosity and dilation, hemorrhage, exudates, cotton-wool lesions, and absence of the central excavation.
- Chronic optic disc changes include: sparse hemorrhages and exudates, capillary telangiectasis, occipital shunt vessels, rarefaction of the capillary network, and cotton-wool lesions on the optic disc.
- Optic atrophy develops later in only 50% of cases.

Fluorescein Angiography

- Premature leakage of the dye from the dilated capillaries on the optic disc takes place.
- In the arteriovenous phase, diffuse hyperfluorescence develops due to leakage from the prepapillary capillaries.
- In the late phase, diffuse hyperfluorescence continues to be visible.
- A flecked, finely granulated hyperfluorescence in the late phase is typical of older papilledema.

Diagnosis and Treatment

- The diagnosis is based on the case history, combined with the bilateral optic disc findings. It is typical to find that the vessels at the edge of the optic disc are covered by the accumulated axons.
- An enlarged blind spot can be seen in the visual field; later, deficits can mostly be found in the inferior and nasal area.
- Widened optic nerve sheaths are recognizable with ultrasound.
- Cranial computed tomography and a neurological examination should be carried out for further clarification of bilateral optic disc edema.
- In patients with unilateral optic disc edema, computed tomography and/or magnetic resonance imaging of the orbits using contrast are indicated.
- Neurological and neurosurgical treatment of the underlying disease is usually carried out. It is important to avoid any factors that might increase intracranial pressure. If this occurs, osmotherapy or corticosteroid therapy may be necessary.
- Diuretics are recommended for pseudotumor cerebri.
- Papilledema resolves 6–10 weeks after the intracranial pressure is reduced.

References

Frisen L. Swelling of the optic nerve head: a staging scheme. J Neurol Neurosurg Psychiatry 1982;45:13–8.

Glaser JS. Topical diagnosis: the optic nerve. In: Tasman W, Jaeger EA, eds. Duane's clinical ophthalmology. New York: Lippincott Williams and Wilkins, 1999: 50–7.

Tso MO, Hayreh SS. Optic disc edema in raised intracranial pressure, 3: a pathologic study of experimental papilledema. Arch Ophthalmol 1977;95:1448–57.

Tso MO, Hayreh SS. Optic disc edema in raised intracranial pressure, 4: axoplasmic transport in experimental papilledema. Arch Ophthalmol 1977;95:1458–62.

White WN, Corbett J, Wall M. Raised intracranial pressure. In: Rosen ES, Thompson HS, Cumming WJ, Eustace P, eds. Neuroophthalmology. London: Mosby, 1998: 21.1–21.12.

10

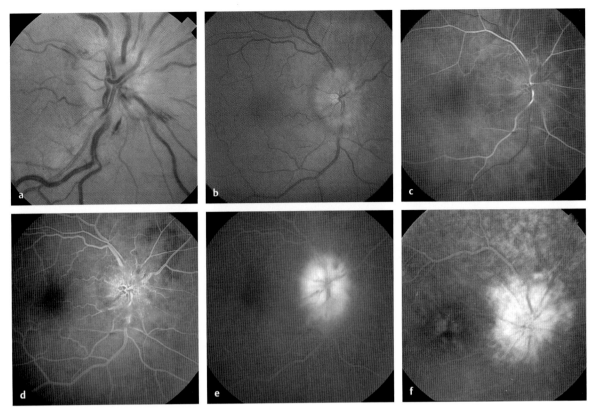

Fig. 10.4a–f Papilledema

a Color photograph. There is a prominent and irregular optic disc, and the excavation has disappeared. Dilation of the vessels and stripe-shaped hemorrhages can be seen.

b Color photograph. There is a prominent and irregular optic disc, and the excavation has disappeared. Rarefaction of the capillary network on the optic disc, with a circular halo, and cotton-wool lesions within the optic disc are visible.

c Early phase. Premature leakage of the dye from the dilated capillaries can be observed on the optic disc.

d Arteriovenous phase. Diffuse leakage from the prepapillary capillaries.

e Late phase. Diffuse hyperfluorescence, and the optic disc has indistinct borders.

f Late phase. Flecked, finely granulated hyperfluorescence is typical of long-standing papilledema.

10.5 Combined Juxtapapillary Hamartoma of the Retina and Retinal Pigment Epithelium *Claudia Jandeck*

Epidemiology, Pathophysiology, and Clinical Presentation

- Incidence: some 200 cases have been described in the literature. The condition is usually unilateral.
- The condition can be described as an idiopathic benign pigment epithelial lesion with a juxtapapillary location and finger-shaped infiltration of the retinal pigment epithelium into the sensory retina with reactive gliosis, neovascularization, and dysfunction of the Kuhnt tissue.
- The histological examination shows abnormal accumulation of the normal tissues in specific areas, some of which may show excessive growth, and hyperplasia of the retinal pigment epithelium, glia cells, and blood vessels.
- The lesion affects the optic disc and the surrounding retina.
- Ophthalmoscopy shows a large, slightly prominent, gray-brown lesion with indistinct borders in the optic disc area. The lesion consists of a dark-pigmented external portion with an overlying thickened and semitranslucent gray membrane often with feathery extensions that reach toward the adjacent normal-appearing retina. Many small fine capillaries are recognizable in the tumor.
- The clinical symptoms consist of a reduction in visual acuity by ≤ 0.1 in 40% of cases, strabismus, and metamorphopsia due to contraction of the membrane or occasionally due to subretinal and intraretinal exudations. The exudations may be spontaneously resorbed, leaving behind atrophic changes to the retinal pigment epithelium surrounding the tumor.
- The course is slow and gradual. Choroidal neovascularizations, retinal and vitreous body hemorrhage, and macular holes can occur as complications.

Fluorescein Angiography

- In the early phase, blockage of the background fluorescence takes place in the area of the pigmented areas.
- In the middle phase, a fine network of dilated capillaries and microaneurysms can be seen.
- In the late phase, marked leakage from the dilated and tortuous capillaries develops; the retinal vessels are not altered.

Diagnosis and Treatment

- The diagnosis is generally based on the typical ophthalmoscopic and fluorescence-angiographic findings.
- As the course is only slowly progressive, there is no direct form of therapy; only the complications can be treated.
- Surgical removal of the reactive epiretinal gliosis is difficult, with only a small chance of improving visual acuity.

References

Gass JD. Combined pigment epithelial and retinal hamartoma. In: Gass JD, ed. Stereoscopic atlas of macular diseases: diagnosis and treatment, 4th ed. St. Louis: Mosby, 1997: 824–7.

Laqua H, Wessing A. Congenital retino-pigment epithelial malformation, previously described as hamartoma. Am J Ophthalmol 1979;87:34–42.

Schachat AP, Shields JA, Fine SL, et al. Combined hamartomas of the retina and retinal pigment epithelium. Ophthalmology 1984;91:1609–15.

Verma L, Venkatesh P, Lakshmaiah CN, Tewari HK. Combined hamartoma of the retina and retinal pigment epithelium with full thickness retinal hole and without retinoschisis. Ophthalmic Surg Lasers 2000;31:423–6.

10

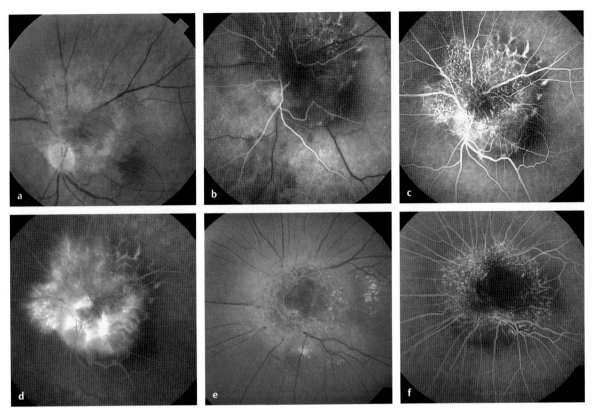

Fig. 10.**5a–f   Combined juxtapapillary hamartoma of the retina and retinal pigment epithelium**

a Color photograph. There is a large, slightly prominent, gray-brown lesion with indistinct borders in the optic disc area.

b Early phase. Blockage of the background fluorescence in the region of the pigmented areas.

c Arteriovenous phase. Microaneurysms and a fine network of abnormal, dilated capillaries with leakage are visible. The network covers the whole tumor.

d Late phase. Marked diffuse leakage from the dilated and tortuous vessels. The retinal vessels are impervious to fluorescein.

e Color photograph. There is a slight, prominent, brownish lesion with indistinct borders in the region of the optic disc.

f Middle phase. Numerous microaneurysms, dilated capillaries with leakage. There is a blockage in the area of the brownish changes.

10

10.6 Peripapillary Choroidal Neovascularizations   *Claudia Jandeck*

Epidemiology, Pathophysiology, and Clinical Presentation

- There are many different possible causes for the development of peripapillary choroidal neovascularizations (CNV). The most common are age-related macular degeneration, peripapillary choroiditis, presumed ocular histoplasmosis syndrome, hyaline drusen in the region of the optic disc, congenital optic disc anomalies, and angioid streaks.
- Etiologically, there are peripapillary changes and defects in Bruch membrane.
- The growth of a peripapillary choroidal neovascularization is mainly asymptomatic and does not affect visual acuity. Reduced visual acuity develops with secondary involvement of the fovea.
- Enlargement of the blind spot can be detected in the visual field, along with a paracentral scotoma.
- The course of peripapillary choroidal neovascularization can remain static for a long time. Due to the rareness of the condition, there are no definitive data regarding the natural course of the disease or the frequency of visual acuity loss.
- Subsequent possible changes include: cystoid macular edema, retinal degeneration over the lesion, hemorrhoidal detachment of the retinal pigment epithelium, exudative retinal detachment, and vitreous body hemorrhage.

Fluorescein Angiography

- The diagnosis of peripapillary choroidal neovascularization is established with fluorescein angiography.
- Mild leakage develops in the affected areas in the early phase.
- Marked leakage with indistinct borders is seen in the late phase.

Diagnosis and Treatment

- The diagnosis is based on ophthalmoscopy and fluorescein angiography.
- Fluorescein angiography makes it possible to define the borders and activity of the choroidal neovascularization as well as the accompanying subretinal changes.
- There are at present no conclusive and definitive studies on the indications for treatment. Depending on the symptoms laser coagulation should be considered, depending on the growth and position of the choroidal neovascularization. Subretinal surgery and photodynamic therapy have recently been reported as alternative treatments, but conclusive recommendations are not yet possible.

References

Bains HS, Patel MR, Singh H, et al. Surgical treatment of extensive peripapillary choroidal neovascularization in elderly patients. Retina 2003;23:469–74.

Browning DJ, Fraser CM. Ocular conditions associated with peripapillary subretinal neovascularization, their relative frequencies, and associated outcomes. Ophthalmology 2005;112:1054–61.

Flaxel CJ, Bird AC, Hamilton AM, Gregor ZJ. Partial laser ablation of massive peripapillary subretinal neovascularization. Ophthalmology 1996;103:1250–9.

Kokame GT, Yamamoka S. Subretinal surgery for peripapillary subretinal neovascular membranes. Retina 2005;25:564–9.

Lopez PF, Green WR. Peripapillary subretinal neovascularization: a review. Retina 1992;12:147–71.

Rosenblatt BJ, Shah GK, Blinder K. Photodynamic therapy with verteporfin for peripapillary choroidal neovascularization. Retina 2005;25:33–7.

10

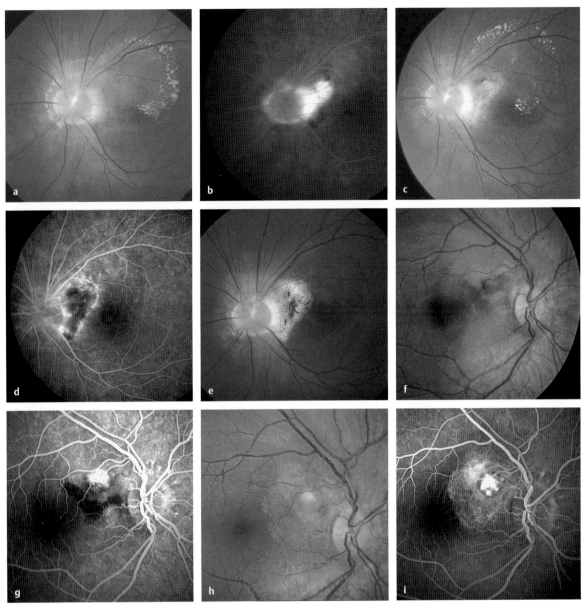

Fig. 10.6a–i Peripapillary choroidal neovascularizations

a Color photograph. A peripapillary choroidal neovascularization with clear exudates developed in the area of the temporal upper vessel arcade; visual acuity 0.02.

b Late phase. Leakage with indistinct borders in the area of the choroidal neovascularization.

c Color photograph. Same patient as in **a**, 3 months later. After laser coagulation of the choroidal neovascularization, there is minor regression of the secondary exudations; visual acuity has improved to 0.1.

d Arteriovenous phase. Leakage at the border of the laser scar, but no recurrence.

e Color photograph. The same patient as in **a**, 18 months later. There is a laser coagulation scar temporal to the optic disc, with no more residual exudate. Visual acuity is 0.2.

f Color photograph. This 10-year-old patient had a peripapillary choroidal neovascularization with subretinal hemorrhage; visual acuity 1.0.

g Arteriovenous phase. Leakage with blurred borders in the region of the choroidal neovascularization, and blockage in the area of the hemorrhage.

h Color photograph. The same patient as in **f** 2 years later, with no therapeutic intervention. The peripapillary choroidal neovascularization is surrounded by pigment epithelial defects; visual acuity 1.0.

i Arteriovenous phase. There is hyperfluorescence in the area of the pigment epithelial defect and leakage in the area of the choroidal neovascularization.

10

Index

Page references in **bold type** refer to illustrations.